You Won't Believe It's Salt-Free!

You Won't Believe It's
SALT-FREE!

125 Heart-Healthy, Low-Sodium
and No-Sodium Recipes Using
Flavorful Spice Blends

ROBYN WEBB

Da Capo
LIFE
LONG

A Member of the Perseus Books Group

Book design by Timm Bryson
Cataloging-in-Publication data for this book is available from the Library of Congress.

First Da Capo Press edition 2012
ISBN: 978-0-7382-1556-3 (paperback)

Published by Da Capo Press
A Member of the Perseus Books Group
www.dacapopress.com

Da Capo Press books are available at special discounts for bulk purchases in the U.S. by corporations, institutions, and other organizations. For more information, please contact the Special Markets Department at the Perseus Books Group, 2300 Chestnut Street, Suite 200, Philadelphia, PA, 19103, or call (800) 810-4145, ext. 5000, or e-mail special.markets@perseusbooks.com.

10 9 8 7 6 5 4 3 2 1

TO MY MOTHER RUTH

the original salt-free pioneer who knew
early on that reducing her salt intake
would lead to a longer and healthier life—
she's eighty-eight years young!

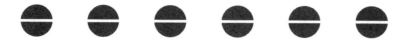

Contents

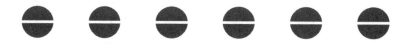

Introduction: The Truth About Salt

As a nutritionist, I've seen just about every type of food "vice" there is, and then some. Some of my clients have a penchant for sugar; others love creamy, fatty foods. Many crave salt and lots of it. And we nutritionists are not exactly exempt from these cravings. I always chuckle when my clients think I'm picture-perfect healthy when it comes to the foods I choose to eat. While much of my daily diet is comprised of healthful foods, my little "secret" is my desire for salt. I have always cooked with it, albeit preferring a tasty kosher salt or sea salt over the bland table variety. Give me foods that are high in sodium—olives, capers, anchovies, full-sodium soy sauce— and I'm in taste heaven!

As a health professional, I knew I had to break my salt vice. Consuming too much salt puts us at risk for many health conditions, as I'll explain. But as a culinary professional, I wondered—could I *really* make the flavors of food come together without a grain of salt? When the opportunity to produce a cookbook of low-sodium fare arose, I took it. And after hours of creating these scrumptious dishes, I'm thrilled to tell you that you can make meals full of flavor but without the salt! All you need are the right combinations of herbs and spices.

With these easy recipes, not only can you skip the salt, you'll truly begin to appreciate a whole new world of flavorful and wonderfully aromatic herbs and spices. The effect on my team of recipe testers was profound as well. Many of them could not believe that these delicious recipes did not have a salt shaker in sight. Now these former "salt junkies" have become herb and spice aficionados.

THE TRUTH ABOUT SALT, A.K.A. SODIUM

Although sodium is one of the many minerals we must consume on a daily basis to keep our body's basic functions operating, we typically consume significantly more than we need. Consider the following: Our body requires anywhere from 250 to 500 milligrams of sodium a day to keep nerves and muscles working and ensure our cells have the right amount of water in them. Government and health organization guidelines have established 2,300 milligrams as the maximum recommended daily limit—and for anyone with hypertension or who is over the age of forty, no more than 1,500 milligrams. Meanwhile, the average American takes in anywhere from 3,400 to 3,700 milligrams of sodium per day! That certainly helps explain why 65 million Americans currently live with hypertension (high blood pressure), while another 45 million walk around with prehypertension. We are even starting to see children as young as three years old with hypertension (almost 2 million hypertension cases involve those age eighteen or younger).

Consuming too much salt is problematic for a variety of reasons. Approximately one-third of Americans are considered "sodium sensitive," meaning that excessive sodium intake negatively affects their blood pressure. High blood pressure readings are bad news, because they are a pretty good predictor of cardiovascular disease risk: when our blood pressure rises, our blood vessels take a significant hit. They are over-worked, and therefore more prone to bursting. Additionally, all the strain they endure can create tiny lesions that can rapidly become a home for plaque and cholesterol to accumulate. No wonder research has established that cardiovascular disease risk doubles for every 10-point increase in diastolic blood pressure (the bottom number) and every 20-point increase in systolic blood pressure (the top number).

One of the most disturbing characteristics of high blood pressure is that it is mostly symptom-free; only in extreme cases do people "not feel well." This is why it is important to not only regularly consult a doctor but also to keep tabs on your sodium intake; you may feel just fine, while your blood vessels and heart are literally fighting for their lives—and yours—on a daily basis.

It's not just heart health that is affected by damaged arteries. High blood pressure is a risk factor for other conditions having to do with impaired blood flow, from impotence and vascular dementia to blurry vision and kidney failure. In the case of pregnant women, high blood pressure is harmful to them and to the fetus they carry, as it can cause premature delivery as well as low birth weight. These are just some examples of why keeping the salt habit in check is so important.

Let's go back to that "sodium sensitive" business. Some people assume that if they are among the two-thirds of the population that is not sodium-sensitive and don't have high blood pressure, then they don't have to worry one bit. Think again.

High intake of sodium in the diet can leach calcium from bones, and can therefore increase one's risk of—and speed up—osteoporosis. It is also important to point out that diets high in sodium tend to be low in other key minerals, such as potassium and magnesium. You see, the more processed a food is, the higher its sodium content and lower its potassium content. This is problematic because potassium plays a very important role, not only in heart health, but also in blood pressure regulation. High-sodium foods also tend to be low in healthful minerals such as manganese and magnesium. So, even if one is not sensitive to the blood-pressure raising effects of sodium, a high-sodium diet lacks many health-promoting nutrients.

Here's the good news. Hypertension can be treated—and, more important, prevented—by eating a healthful diet low in sodium and high in nutrient-rich whole foods. It is the goal of this book to broaden your taste buds to try all kinds of herbs and spices as a delicious replacement for salt. From simple family dinners to recipes using exotic herbs and spices, there is something for everyone's palate. Once you experiment beyond the salt shaker, your health will improve and your cooking will, too!

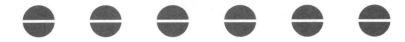

Secrets of Salt-Free Cooking

The recipes in this book will show you how to:

- add maximum flavor without a lot of fuss through the use of already prepared salt-free herb and spice blends
- use basic, familiar fresh herbs to bolster the flavor of dishes in place of salt
- take advantage of less commonly used (but available) and highly flavorful aromatic whole spices and exotic herbs

ABOUT THE SALT-FREE BLENDS USED IN THESE RECIPES

One of the easiest ways to cut down or eliminate the salt shaker is to use salt-free herb and spice blends. A majority of the recipes in this book are best using these convenient and flavorful seasonings, which you can find at most any supermarket. Salt-free herb and spice blends serve as an excellent introduction to no/low-sodium cooking. All it takes is a few good shakes of these mixtures and you can replace the sodium in most any dish.

While talking with many of my clients, I found that they didn't know how to use salt-free seasonings to maximize flavor in their cooking. They didn't know how much or how little to use, or which salt-free blends should be used with what foods. They basically felt that if they had some guidance and a collection of easy recipes to use as a springboard, they would be able to reduce their sodium intake with little effort. As a result, I felt it was important to include readily available blended seasonings in this book.

In choosing which salt-free blends to include, I scoured the many companies that produce them. Ultimately, I chose seven of the Mrs. Dash® line of salt-free seasonings. I found that the flavors were well balanced and they really did eliminate the need for salt. The seven Mrs. Dash blends used in this book are:

- Lemon Pepper
- Southwest Chipotle
- Italian Medley (I refer to that as Italian seasoning in these recipes)
- Garlic & Herb
- Original Blend (I refer to that as all-purpose seasoning in these recipes)
- Caribbean Citrus
- Chicken Grilling Blend

These seven choices reflect my quest to create recipes that give an assertive punch of flavor without being overwhelming. When you have relied on salt for so long to solely carry flavor, a bold substitute has to be skillfully used. If you have your own favorite salt-free seasoning in any of the above flavors, feel free to substitute yours in the recipes. If we performed a side-by-side comparison of my recipes prepared with the Mrs. Dash blends and with your favorites, there might be some variation in taste, but I'm confident the results would be just as delicious.

I also chose these seven blends for other reasons. Dried spices are best when used within one year of purchase. If you stock up on too many seasoning blends, chances are the seldom-used ones will go to waste. The flavorings I chose to use for this book are used over and over again so they will stay fresh. For instance, the Southwestern Chipotle seasoning works beautifully in everything from Bread Dips (page 27) to Southwestern Coleslaw (page 104) to Chocolate Chile Nut Meringues (really, this spice blend is a winner in a cookie! page 144). There's nothing more frustrating than purchasing dried spices, not knowing what to do with them, and then having them go to waste. It is my goal that you will use what you buy across a variety of dishes, from appetizers through desserts.

There is one more blend I particularly like and use quite a bit of in this book: tandoori-style seasoning. My preference is the blend sold by another favorite company, Penzeys, which has an online catalog as well as its own stores located in the Midwest and along the East Coast. Penzeys fabulous Tandoori Seasoning is a mixture of coriander, cumin, sweet paprika, garlic, ginger, cardamom, and saffron. The Penzeys catalog is well worth a review and this company, too, like Mrs. Dash, offers a variety of other salt-free seasonings. To order, go to www.penzeys.com or call 1-800-741-7787. If you live near a Penzeys store, I highly recommend you pay it a visit. The store is heaven "scent"! Another tandoori seasoning I used in testing the recipes comes from Dean and Deluca. Their beautiful Tandoori Blend can also be ordered online at www.deandeluca.com, or visit one of their elegant stores.

MAKE-IT-YOURSELF BLENDS

There may be times that you run out of a particular blend or it may be temporarily unavailable, so I've developed a few blends you can make from scratch:

Lemon Pepper: Make your own Lemon Pepper seasoning by combining 1 teaspoon of grated fresh lemon zest and ¼ teaspoon of freshly ground black pepper. Commercially prepared Lemon Pepper seasoning is more complex than this, but this quickie homemade mix is great in a pinch.

Caribbean Blend: Make your own Caribbean Citrus seasoning by combining 1 ½ tablespoons of ground allspice, 3 tablespoons of minced fresh thyme leaves, 1 ½ teaspoons of sweet paprika, 1 teaspoon of orange zest, ⅛ teaspoon of ground cloves, and ⅛ teaspoon of ground nutmeg.

Tandoori Blend: Make your own tandoori-style seasoning from scratch by combining 1 teaspoon of ground coriander, 1 teaspoon of ground cumin, 1 teaspoon of sweet paprika, ½ teaspoon of garlic powder, ¼ teaspoon of ground ginger, ⅛ teaspoon of ground cardamom, and a pinch of crumbled saffron.

TIPS FOR KEEPING DRIED HERBS AND SPICES FRESH

- Use herbs, spices, and blends within one year of purchase. After a year, aromatic oils diminish and flavor is flat. Keep caps and lids sealed tight to prevent air and moisture from seeping in.
- Keep herbs, spices, and blends away from heat (even away from the refrigerator, as it is an appliance that gives off heat). The best place to store them is in a kitchen drawer so you can see at a glance what you have and when it's time to replenish.
- Don't sprinkle herbs, spices, or blends straight from the bottle over foods while they are cooking. Steam that rises into the bottle can dampen and spoil the life of the seasonings.
- To release even more flavor from blends, try rubbing them between your fingers before adding to your recipe. This releases more of the aromatic oils.
- If you find you are not using particular dried herb and spice blends fast enough, offer to share your blends with friends and neighbors.

BASIC FRESH HERBS

I can't imagine a pesto without fresh basil or a mint julep without the mint! Fresh herbs really tie a recipe together with their clean, heady aromas and flavors. Everything from zingy rosemary to subtle parsley, when used by the pinch or by the handful, can really elevate a dish to new heights.

I'm often amazed at just how many people do not use fresh herbs at all and rely solely on salt and pepper to carry all the flavor in a dish. Such a big mistake! They reason that they just don't know which herb to add to which food, or believe herbs are too complicated to use. Both concerns are very real and I recommend starting with the basic herbs and spices, to overcome any fears. The following are the herbs and spices that you'll find used in the recipes in this book:

Basil: One of the most often used herbs is basil. It has a very nice undertone of both cloves and licorice. It is one of the easiest to grow yourself and is amazingly versatile. You really can't go wrong in adding it to most soups, sandwiches, salads, main dishes, and even dessert (lemon basil is perfect in fruit salads). What I love most about basil is that there are so many ways you can cut it.

- You can leave basil whole and use it as another green in your favorite salad. Whole leaves paired with dark greens in a salad that also contains tomatoes work extremely well.
- Slice basil into a chiffonade or shred it; it looks lovely scattered over a bowl of soup or as a garnish for fish or chicken entrées.
- When chopped into bits, basil permeates a lovely homemade tomato sauce, or add it to jarred tomato sauce for a kick.

Try all of basil's cousins if you can; purple ruffle basil is beautiful in salads, lemon basil is great in drinks and desserts, and Thai basil is of course important in Thai-inspired dishes such as curries. In addition to growing different kinds of basil yourself, many groceries and supermarkets have several varieties available all year long.

Chives: Sprightly and slightly onionlike in flavor, chives are a very delicate herb. Chives won't deliver a powerful punch when used alone in a recipe, but that's okay if you want a subtle onion flavor. When chives are paired with onions in a dish, you can create deep, multidimensional flavor. Heat really destroys the flavor of chives, so they are best used in cold dishes or as a garnish to hot foods. I really love the garlic chive variety; it's a flatter and wider herb that packs even more flavor than its skinny cousin.

Cilantro: This is one of those herbs that people tend to feel strongly about—many love it, others loathe it! Cilantro is the leaf of the coriander plant and some people label cilantro as coriander. Others call it Chinese parsley. But don't get flat-leaf parsley and cilantro confused. Although they look similar, cilantro has a distinctive pungent flavor with a faint taste of anise, while parsley is much milder.

When you first start using cilantro, use it sparingly. It's terrific in salsa and soups, particularly bean soups. It pairs well with dried spices such as cumin, turmeric, and paprika, and it goes well with dishes that include lime or lemon and curry dishes. To see if you like the taste of fresh cilantro in your food, separate a small portion of your dish from the rest, add the cilantro, and taste. Because it has such an assertive flavor, see if it suits your palate before adding too much.

Mint: Just a sprinkle of chopped fresh mint and a pinch of lemon zest is all that is needed to liven up fresh peas. This is one of my very favorite herbs. Who can resist its cool-as-an-ocean-breeze taste? I got hooked on fresh mint while traveling throughout the Middle East and I just can't enough of its fresh, sweet flavor. Spearmint is the preferred form of mint over its darker cousin peppermint.

Use mint when you want a cooling effect in your dishes. It's fairly bold, so often it doesn't need to be paired with other herbs or spices. Mint brings out the sweetness of ice cream and other frozen treats and is refreshing in drinks from lemonade to flavored iced teas. It's one of the herbs I prefer only in its fresh form. Like basil, it has some fabulous cousins such as orange, grapefruit, ginger, lemon, and my favorite, chocolate mint.

Oregano: What would Mediterranean cooking be without potent oregano? Oregano grows wild in the mountains of Greece and Italy. It gives vinaigrettes; fish, poultry, and meat dishes; sauces; and soups the rich, heady aroma and flavor we associate with these countries' cuisines. It's bold and more assertive than basil, another Mediterranean herb, so be judicious when first experimenting with oregano. It's one of those herbs that makes a pretty garnish; use the entire branch of leaves whole. It also dries well; just tie the branches together and hang in a well-ventilated, dry area until dry to the touch.

Oregano has a cousin called marjoram. Marjoram is milder than oregano and is perfect when you want a sweeter, milder oregano-like taste. They look very similar so be sure you know what you are buying.

Parsley: If there is only one fresh herb you add to your cooking, I say, make it parsley. You'll be amazed at the difference a simple parsley garnish can make; it brightens up and finishes the look of an entire dish. It's one of those herbs that you can't go wrong with by adding it to practically everything. I call parsley the "cooperative" herb; it's mild and gives other ingredients a chance to come through. I much prefer flat-leafed parsley to the curly variety, because it has much more flavor and stands up better to heat.

One of the easiest ways to use parsley is to combine it with citrus zest and sprinkle it over everything from soups to salads to main dishes. So next time, don't ignore the directions for a parsley garnish; it can turn a simple dish into something extraordinary.

Rosemary: Talk about a gutsy herb! I love rosemary's lemony, pinelike flavor. It holds its strong, forward flavor, so use it in small quantities to start; use too much and your dish just might end up tasting medicinal. I recommend pairing rosemary with a milder herb such as parsley or thyme to give balance to the overall dish.

Thyme: Ah, versatile thyme. It has a vibrant, yet slightly subtle mint lemon flavor that goes well with so many dishes. It has a natural affinity for lamb, tomatoes, and peas, but I add it to so many foods with great results. Because thyme is strong but not overwhelming, it actually pairs well with other herbs and does well in combinations so that the flavor does not become one-dimensional. Its cousin lemon thyme is really special and if you grow it or buy it, try it in iced teas and fruit desserts.

TIPS FOR PURCHASING AND STORING FRESH HERBS

I realize that not everyone wants to or can grow fresh herbs. Fortunately you can almost always purchase fresh and dried basic herbs and spices at your local grocery store or market. These tips will ensure you get the freshest herbs possible.

- Herb packaging may vary: loose, in a box, tied in a bundle, or still growing in a pot. Look for herbs with vibrant color and a fresh aroma. Avoid brown, black, or yellowing herbs, limp herbs, or those that smell damp or off in any way.
- There are hardy herbs and more delicate ones. Rosemary is an example of a hardy herb and it will stay fresh and fragrant for about a week in the refrigerator. Tender herbs such as basil, cilantro, and parsley need a little bit more attention. Place these herbs bouquet style in a jar of water covering about 1 inch of the stem. Cover with a plastic bag to enclose the herbs in the glass jar, and change the water every other day.
- To keep herbs looking their best, when you get them home, remove any fasteners. Because the roots draw

moisture from the leaves, trim the root ends and lower parts of the stem to prevent the herb from wilting.

- Wrap trimmed herbs loosely in damp paper towels. Do not wash herbs until you are ready to use them because excess moisture shortens their shelf life in the refrigerator.
- Store your herbs in the warmest part of the refrigerator, usually a top shelf. Don't store herbs in the produce bins of your refrigerator; it is way too cold.
- When you are ready to wash your herbs, put them in a large bowl of cool water and just swish them around to release any dirt. Lift out the herbs with your hands or a sieve. Spin dry them in a salad spinner or roll them up in a clean towel to dry them.

GROWING HERBS

Volumes have been written on how to grow herbs, but if you consider yourself born without a green thumb, herbs just might be the plants for you! Growing them is really simple and does not require a degree in botany.

- Start out with just a few. I highly recommend basil, chives, thyme, and rosemary. These grow well with little attention and fuss.
- Herbs need at least five to seven hours of sunshine a day, so take that into account when planning your garden.
- Like flowers, herbs need to be placed in a good soil and need consistent but not excessive watering. The soil should just feel moist.
- To keep your herbs looking full, encourage them to continue growing by snipping off a few leaves every other day. This will prevent the plants from going to seed.
- Each herb has its own special gardening tricks and tips. For best results I recommend you visit your local nursery or scour the numerous websites or books on the subject of growing herbs.

PREPARING FRESH HERBS

A sharp knife is an absolute must for chopping fresh herbs; a dull knife will only crush and bruise them. You may also use a pair of scissors to cut small quantities of herbs; chives in particular cut well with scissors. Another tool I really love to cut herbs with is a mezzaluna. A mezzaluna is a curved blade that chops as you rock it back and forth on a cutting board. It can chop large quantities of herbs quite efficiently and it's available for purchase at most kitchen tool shops.

Chop your herbs as close to the preparation of your recipe as possible. If you have to chop ahead of time, cover the chopped herbs with plastic wrap punctured with a few little holes and refrigerate the herbs.

If you want your overall dish to have a subtle flavor of herbs, consider adding a whole sprig at the beginning of your cooking. Strong herbs such as rosemary and thyme actually do quite well when added early in the cooking process as they mellow very nicely.

If you want your overall dish to have an assertive herb flavor, chop the herbs and add them near the end of the cooking process. You can also use both methods: add herbs at the beginning in the form of a whole sprig and then the same herb chopped at the end of the cooking.

What about the stems? Save tender stems for flavoring stocks. If you grow your own herbs, use the tender stems of cilantro, dill, and parsley; just chop the stems along with the leaves.

For woodier stems such as rosemary or thyme, pull the leaves off in the opposite direction of the way the leaves grow. You should be able to strip them off the stem in one fell swoop. Then chop the leaves.

Woody stems can also be used on the grill instead of wood chips. If your rosemary stems are stiff and long enough, use them to thread on meats and vegetables for kebabs on the grill.

COOKING WITH EXOTIC HERBS AND SPICES

Don't be timid when it comes to branching out of your comfort zone. When you are ready to try some of the more exotic herbs and spices, you will find they will lend such richness and depth to your cooking. You'll never miss the salt when you use some of the ones I have chosen here. And while I call them exotic, putting them into use is so very simple. All of these can be purchased online at Penzeys Spices (www.penzeys.com) or Dean and Deluca (www.deandeluca.com). Also check your local grocer, as many of these flavorings are now available in many grocery stores and markets. Fresh lemongrass, for example is much more readily available in local supermarkets these days. I use many of these exotics in the dessert recipes to give them a special alluring twist on usual fare.

Some of the exotics are dried whole spices, some are ground blends that have been used in a particular culture for centuries, and some are fresh herbs and spices that are used whole. Whole spices and herbs are so easy to use and are the best choice when you want subtle background notes of a particular flavor. Think of whole spices as infusions like teas; the flavor brews gently and permeates a dish with a heady but gentle aroma.

Chinese five-spice powder: This intriguing seasoning is the perfect representation of the Chinese concept of yin and yang (balance in flavors) and is indeed made up of five spices. Which spices are included will vary from blend to blend, but typically it is made of star anise, cloves, cinnamon (cassia; see page 16), Sichuan peppercorns, and ground fennel. The proportion of these spices is often not equal. When you taste Chinese five-spice powder, the first taste is of a strong, deeply rich cinnamon, followed by the remaining spices all balancing on your palate in a warm, inviting crescendo of flavors. That's why I chose to use it in a few of the desserts, as the taste is so unexpected but such a delight.

Try placing Chinese five-spice powder in a shaker container; just set it out on the table to sprinkle over simple foods such as steamed green beans or broccoli. Unusual, I know, but it works! Although Chinese five-spice powder is usually reserved for duck dishes and Asian cuisine, I found it works well beyond these with many more delicious applications.

Cinnamon sticks: As one of the oldest spices known to mankind, anything flavored with cinnamon gets my vote! Cinnamon sticks are not as powerful as ground cinnamon, but provide a subtle flavor that is great in braised dishes and in fruit syrups (see Berries in Ginger Peppercorn Syrup, page 148).

There are actually two types of cinnamon, cassia and Ceylon. Cassia is native to southeast Asia and has a strong, spicy, sweet flavor. Within the category of cassia there are Vietnamese and Chinese cassia, which are the sweetest, and then Korintje, which has less bite with a smoother flavor. Cassia does not have the outer bark removed and is thicker and coarser than Ceylon cinnamon. It is the type of cinnamon used in Chinese five-spice powder (see page 15). Ceylon, or what is referred to as "true" cinnamon, is less sweet and has a citrusy flavor.

I highly recommend you special-order your cinnamon sticks, as they will be more flavorful than those from the grocery store shelf and are well worth purchasing. When you are purchasing ground cinnamon, I also recommend that you sample a variety, from Ceylon to Chinese cassia to Vietnamese. Try them in different recipes and see which kind you like best!

Whole cloves: Cloves are the pink flower buds of the clove tree and are dried in the sun, where they turn a reddish brown. Although traditionally they make their appearance around the holidays to stud a ham or an orange for punch, I love to use cloves way beyond the holiday time. Cloves are great in stews and fruit sauces. They're quite strong, so I don't recommend using cloves all by themselves; they go great with other sweet spices such as nutmeg and cinnamon.

I grind my own cloves in a spice grinder when I need to use this spice in powdered form. The aroma of do-it-yourself ground cloves is so potent you won't quite believe it's cloves, after smelling ground cloves sold in a grocery store.

Crystallized ginger: Ground ginger is used widely and fresh ginger is increasingly familiar, no longer a strange, brown tentacle of a spice. But the use of crystallized ginger in cooking is still new to many people and its warm sweet qualities are too good to pass up. Crystallized ginger is simply fresh ginger slices that have been dried with a sugar coating. While I've included crystallized ginger in the dessert chapter, quite honestly if you mince it up and sprinkle over green salads, add to salad dressings, or top simple steamed green vegetables, your food will pop with flavor. My favorite crystallized ginger to purchase, since it stays so moist, is from The Ginger People (www.gingerpeople.com). If your ginger becomes too hard to chop, add slices to a steamer basket set in a pot with water underneath the steamer. Cover and steam over high heat for just a few minutes and the ginger will become pliable again!

Garam masala: One of the teaching tools I use to expose my clients to new culinary delights is to have them partake in blind aroma tests of unusual herbs and spices. I like to see if they would try some of the sumptuous blends based on smell alone. The one that brings the most oohs and aahs is garam masala. This Indian mixture is the general name for a family of spices that can be at once hot with the inclusion of chile and cloves, and aromatic with mace, cinnamon, and cardamom. Other ingredients may also include ground coriander, peppercorns, ginger, and nutmeg. As with Chinese five-spice powder, don't limit your use to the country of origin's recipes. I often just add a sprinkle of garam masala to cooked carrots or spinach and the food goes from ho-hum to spectacular. There are many masalas; garam masala is the most familiar and the most readily available in the United States.

Herbes de Provence: Imagine a blend so potent that it almost can carry you to another place and time. This heady mixture of savory, fennel, basil, thyme, and sometimes lavender transports me to my favorite region in the world: Southern France. Every time I open my little pot of herbes de Provence, visions of sunny fields, olive trees, and rock hillsides come to mind. No wonder using this fabulous blend makes your food taste so special.

Herbes de Provence is best with grilled foods. Never add it to foods after they have been cooked; it needs a bit of cooking to open up all the flavors. You don't have to make a special trip across the ocean to enjoy herbes de Provence; it's just a click away through mail order!

Kaffir lime leaves: When I was first visited Thailand, I couldn't discern where the lovely aroma was coming from in my seemingly plain rice dish. A server graciously said it was something called Kaffir lime leaf that was perfuming my grain. He then brought out from the kitchen a bumpy looking lime and presented it as if it were the crown jewel of Thailand. I suppose Kaffir lime and its leaves could be considered royalty in Thai cooking and it also works beautifully in Asian-influenced foods.

Kaffir lime leaves are actually two leaves attached together to form somewhat of a figure eight. The leaves are either sliced and added to soups, curries, and rice dishes, or used whole to infuse flavor into a dish. They can be found fresh or frozen at Asian markets. If you cannot locate Kaffir lime leaf, you may substitute 1 tablespoon of lime zest for six Kaffir lime leaves. I didn't use Kaffir lime leaf extensively in this book, but one of my favorite ways to use it easily is to add whole leaves along with pieces of lemongrass and slices of ginger to a pot of chicken broth and simmer for 20 to 30 minutes. The result is a beautiful lemon ginger broth that is perfect on a cold, wintry day.

Peppercorns: As far as I am concerned, the shakers for salt and pepper should be reversed: the shaker with more holes should contain pepper rather than salt. I can't imagine preparing most dishes without a good grind of pepper. With so many great varieties, pepper, not salt, should be the spice of choice on the dinner table.

The finest peppercorn is called Tellicherry, a large, mature, well-developed pepper flavor. But branch out and use white peppercorns known for their rich, almost winey and somewhat hot flavor. I've used fresh peppercorns, whole and cracked, in several of the dishes in this book and I think you will agree it's wise to have a full supply of peppercorns available at your kitchen fingertips.

I always start with whole peppercorns and crack the peppercorns using a spice grinder. I also have placed peppercorns in a plastic bag and crushed them using a large cast-iron skillet. For table service, my favorite pepper mill comes from the Penzeys catalog. It's called Zassenhaus and in my opinion, it's one of the finest on the market today. It produces uniform particle size at every setting and never cranks out "pepper dust"!

Saffron: There is no confusing saffron with turmeric, two yellow spices often erroneously thought to be interchangeable in recipes. Saffron is from the crocus family, whereas turmeric is from the pepper family, with a much stronger flavor. Saffron is the soft, beautifully flavored spice that is worth using when recipes call for it. It's actually the stigma of the crocus flower and it is handpicked. It's always been the most expensive spice by weight. But by use, saffron really isn't that expensive because a little goes such a long way. Always use saffron threads, not powdered saffron as it is inferior and is often cut with the more peppery and gingery flavor of turmeric.

Keep saffron well protected in a glass container away from light, air, and moisture.

Star anise: As one of the most beautiful and fragrant spices in the world, star anise packs a wallop of flavor. The star-shaped spice is the fruit of the native Chinese evergreens and has a stronger flavor than typical anise. I've used star anise whole in this book, but be aware it is very strong. It's a flavor I love, but broken or powered star anise is also available if you like things more tempered. Try adding a whole star anise to your next pot of hot tea; it will transform it into a fragrant soothing cup of warmth.

OTHER INGREDIENTS TO ENHANCE FLAVOR WITHOUT ADDED SALT

Citrus: I wouldn't go as far as to claim that using citrus juices and citrus zest exactly mimics the taste of salt. Salt is salt and citrus is, well, citrus. But the reason you see lots of citrus juice and zest in my recipes is that it provides a bright, sprightly flavor. Most vegetables, for instance, can be dramatically improved with just a squeeze of fresh lemon or lime and a little grated zest. Always use fresh juice, never frozen or bottled, and fresh zest that you grate yourself. It makes little sense to accept anything less than fresh when the goal is to get the best flavor from your food. While available year-round, when buying, make sure that lemons, limes, and oranges feel heavy for their size and are uniform in color with no evidence of bruising or browning.

Nuts and Seeds: While nuts and seeds are foods, not spices or herbs, I use the unsalted ones extensively in my recipes to give dishes a toasty flavor. The texture of nuts is very pleasing to the palate, and by using a variety of nuts and seeds you will excite other parts of your taste receptors rather than relying on salt. And of course nuts and seeds provide great quality nutrition: monounsaturated fat, vitamin E, fiber, calcium, and more. In quantity, nuts and seeds can be high in fat and calories; however, I use them in small amounts to make a dish exciting without causing calorie and fat overload.

The way to store nuts and seeds for best freshness is in the freezer and to use what you need a little at a time. To toast all the nuts and seeds in the recipes, simple add the quantity to a dry skillet (no need for oil) and shake over medium heat until the nuts or seeds are lightly browned, watching very carefully that you do not burn them. Always toast your nuts or seeds as directed in the recipe, as raw nuts and seeds provide little flavor.

Best-quality produce: If your goal is to lower the sodium content of your recipes, then you must start with the best-quality produce you can find. When you have the ripest, juiciest tomatoes, salt is unnecessary. You will be able to taste the naturally sweet notes in a high-quality carrot or head of broccoli with just a sprinkle of lemon pepper seasoning; these vegetables will not need salt to bring out their flavor. Try to frequent your local farmers' markets where the fruits and vegetables were probably picked that morning. Shop at smaller supermarkets, where inventory control may be better and they purchase from local vendors. And if you've got a bit of land or some wide pots, why not grow a few tomatoes or some cucumbers of your own? I guarantee that your salt shaker will become obsolete when your produce is top notch.

Avoid salt substitutes: Too often for my taste, people will merely use a salt substitute in place of salt. Truthfully, I find these substitutes very insipid. By replacing salt with one of the many salt substitutes, your food may be lower in overall sodium content, but your food will generally taste off or bitter. Salt substitutes can give food an unpleasant metallic taste. Restricting yourself to the use of these also prevents you from ever experimenting with herbs and spices, the true flavor punch of all the recipes in this book!

SODIUM CONTENT OF RECIPES IN THIS BOOK

The recipes in this book have no added salt, but some foods naturally contain low levels of sodium. I've set the sodium limit of any recipe in this book to 200 mg per serving; in fact, many of the recipes fall below that figure.

The nutritional analyses for the recipes in this book include naturally occurring sodium from fresh produce such as tomatoes, celery, and carrots. Naturally occurring sodium provides other essential nutrients and contributes to overall sodium–potassium balance.

Presently, products sold on grocery store shelves require 140 mg or less per serving to be considered low sodium. You would be hard-pressed to find delicious prepackaged food with 200 mg per serving; most prepackaged foods go well beyond that figure. The bottom line is if you can prepare a recipe at home that gives your taste buds a needed change from high sodium content and hits the ceiling of 200 mg of sodium per serving, while maintaining bold flavor, I consider this a win-win, and I think you will, too!

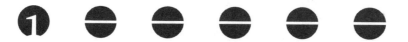

Starters

Lemon Pepper Shrimp Skewer with Grape Tomato Relish

8 SERVINGS/SERVING SIZE: 1 SKEWER, ¼ CUP OF RELISH

PREPARATION TIME: 8 MINUTES

COOK TIME: 16 MINUTES

A large shrimp bowl is nice to serve to guests, and here's a way to offer something unique. Beautifully grilled shrimp with a slight crunchy crust from Lemon Pepper seasoning are paired with basil, lemon juice, and lemon zest–infused grape tomato relish. Yes, this is a bit more interesting than the common shrimp bowl.

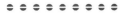

BASIC NUTRITIONAL VALUES

Calories 85
  Calories from Fat 45
Total Fat 5.0 g
  Saturated Fat 1.0 g
  Trans Fat 0 g
Cholesterol 45 mg
Sodium 40 mg
Total Carbohydrate 3 g
  Dietary Fiber 1 g
  Sugars 1 g
Protein 6 g

Grape Tomato Relish

1 cup finely chopped grape tomatoes
½ small red onion, minced
½ large red bell pepper, seeded and minced
2 tablespoons minced fresh basil
2 tablespoons olive oil
1 tablespoon freshly squeezed lemon juice
½ teaspoon grated fresh lemon zest
  Dash of hot sauce

32 large peeled and deveined shrimp, tails on
1 tablespoon salt-free Lemon Pepper seasoning
1 tablespoon olive oil

Garnish
Lemon wedges

1. Soak eight 12-inch wooden skewers in a pan of hot water for 1 hour.

2. Combine all the ingredients for the relish and set aside at room temperature to allow the flavors to develop.

3. Preheat the oven broiler. Line a broiler tray with aluminum foil. Sprinkle the shrimp with the Lemon Pepper seasoning. Thread four shrimp end to end (to keep the shrimp lying flat). Place the shrimp on the broiler tray and drizzle with olive oil.

3. Broil the shrimp, turning once, for a total of 5 to 6 minutes, or until the shrimp turn pink.

4. Serve the shrimp with the relish. Squeeze the lemon wedges over the shrimp if desired.

Roasted Italian Edamame

MAKES 6 CUPS/ SERVING SIZE: ½ CUP

PREPARATION TIME: 5 MINUTES

COOK TIME: 20 TO 30 MINUTES

I call edamame a food chameleon! It takes on different personalities depending on how you prepare it. Sure, you could just cook it up and eat it plain, but why not roast it until it's crispy and add a punchy Italian seasoning. With seven spices and herbs coating each little bean, you won't notice that the salt is missing. These are great little cocktail nibbles.

❋ ❋ ❋ ❋ ❋ ❋ ❋ ❋ ❋

BASIC NUTRITIONAL VALUES

Calories 60
  Calories from Fat 25
Total Fat 3.0 g
  Saturated Fat 0 g
  Trans Fat 0 g
Cholesterol 0 mg
Sodium 0 mg
Total Carbohydrate 5 g
  Dietary Fiber 2 g
  Sugars 1 g
Protein 4 g

Seasoning Mixture

2 teaspoons garlic powder
2 teaspoons onion powder
½ teaspoon dried basil
½ teaspoon dried oregano
½ teaspoon paprika
½ teaspoon sugar
½ teaspoon salt-free Lemon Pepper seasoning

1 (16-ounce) bag frozen shelled edamame
1 tablespoon olive oil

1. Preheat the oven to 400°F. In a bowl, combine the seasoning mixture. Set aside.

2. Defrost the edamame or rinse under cold water until defrosted and pat dry with paper towel.

3. In a large bowl, toss the edamame with the olive oil. Add the seasoning mixture and toss again.

4. Spread the edamame in a single layer on a large nonstick baking sheet. Roast the edamame on the middle rack for 30 to 40 minutes until the edamame is dry to the touch and crunchy, making sure to stir the edamame well every 10 minutes to prevent sticking and burning.

5. Remove the edamame from the oven and let cool for 15 minutes.

6. Store the edamame in a sealed glass container for up to 4 days.

Mushroom Crostini

16 SERVINGS/SERVING SIZE: 2 CROSTINI

PREPARATION TIME: 15 MINUTES

COOK TIME: 25 MINUTES

Feed your guests well before the main course. One whiff of the magnificent aroma of mushrooms accented with Italian seasoning and your guests will think you are a culinary genius.

⊜ ⊜ ⊜ ⊜ ⊜ ⊜ ⊜ ⊜ ⊜

2 ounces dried porcini mushrooms
2 tablespoons olive oil
1 large shallot, minced
2 garlic cloves, minced
¼ cup port wine
1 teaspoon salt-free Italian seasoning
⅛ teaspoon crushed red pepper flakes
5 ounces fresh cremini mushrooms, stemmed and sliced
1 French baguette (8 ounces), cut into thin slices
2 garlic cloves, crushed

Garnishes
Minced fresh parsley
½ teaspoon grated Parmesan cheese per bread slice

1. Place the porcini mushrooms in a medium-size bowl. Pour boiling water over the mushrooms to cover and let stand for 15 to 20 minutes, until soft.

2. Line a strainer with cheesecloth and strain the mushrooms, reserving ½ cup of the soaking liquid. Chop the mushrooms coarsely. Preheat the oven to 400°F.

3. Heat the olive oil in a skillet over medium heat. Add the mushrooms, shallot, and garlic and sauté for 2 minutes. Add the reserved mushroom liquid, port, Italian seasoning, and crushed red pepper flakes. Cover and simmer over low heat for 15 minutes.

4. Uncover the skillet and add the cremini mushrooms. Cook over medium-high heat for 5 to 6 minutes, until the liquid has all evaporated. Keep warm.

5. Place all the bread slices on a large baking sheet. Toast the bread in the 400°F oven just until very lightly browned, 5 to 7 minutes. Remove the bread from the oven and immediately rub the top side of the bread with the crushed garlic. Add a spoonful of the mushroom mixture on top of each bread slice. Garnish with minced parsley and Parmesan cheese.

BASIC NUTRITIONAL VALUES

Calories 80
  Calories from Fat 20
Total Fat 2.5 g
  Saturated Fat 0 g
  Trans Fat 0 g
Cholesterol 0 mg
Sodium 100 mg
Total Carbohydrate 12 g
  Dietary Fiber 1 g
  Sugars 1 g
Protein 3 g

Bread Dips

8 SERVINGS/SERVING SIZE: 1 TABLESPOON

PREPARATION TIME: 5 MINUTES EACH

COOK TIME: 0

These two bread dips will make great conversation starters at your next party. Make them both and see which your guests prefer. (Although it might be a tie; we couldn't decide, either!) Try the Garlic & Herb seasoning with walnut oil and the Southwest Chipotle seasoning with pumpkin oil as variations.

＊＊＊＊＊＊＊＊＊

GARLIC AND HERB DIP

½ cup olive oil
1 tablespoon salt-free Garlic & Herb seasoning
⅛ teaspoon crushed red chili flakes
1 tablespoon good-quality balsamic vinegar

1. Combine the oil, Garlic & Herb seasoning, and chili flakes in a bowl. Pour onto a lipped flat plate. Drizzle the balsamic vinegar in the center of the oil.

BASIC NUTRITIONAL VALUES

Calories 120
  Calories from Fat 125
Total Fat 14.0 g
  Saturated Fat 2.0 g
  Trans Fat 0 g
Cholesterol 0 mg
Sodium 0 mg
Total Carbohydrate 1 g
  Dietary Fiber 0 g
  Sugars 0 g
Protein 0 g

SOUTHWESTERN DIP

½ cup avocado oil or olive oil
1 tablespoon salt-free Southwest Chipotle seasoning
2 teaspoons very finely minced shallot

1. Combine the avocado oil or olive oil, Southwest Chipotle seasoning, and shallot in a bowl. Pour onto a lipped flat plate.

BASIC NUTRITIONAL VALUES

Calories 125
  Calories from Fat 125
Total Fat 14.0 g
  Saturated Fat 1.5 g
  Trans Fat 0 g
Cholesterol 0 mg
Sodium 0 mg
Total Carbohydrate 0 g
  Dietary Fiber 0 g
  Sugars 0 g
Protein 0 g

Cauliflower Crostini

12 SERVINGS/SERVING SIZE: 2 SLICES (2 TABLESPOONS OF CAULIFLOWER MIXTURE PER SLICE)

PREPARATION TIME: 10 MINUTES

COOK TIME: 10 MINUTES

You've heard of tomato crostini, but how about cauliflower crostini? Mashed cooked cauliflower is enhanced with garlic and herbs plus lemon juice and fresh parsley to deliver this light but intriguing appetizer. Try the cauliflower on its own as a side dish.

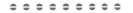

1   medium-size head cauliflower, cut into florets (thick stem and leaves discarded)
3   sprigs fresh thyme
1   sprig fresh rosemary
⅓   cup olive oil
2   tablespoons freshly squeezed lemon juice
2   tablespoons chopped fresh parsley
2   tablespoons salt-free Garlic & Herb seasoning
¼   teaspoon freshly ground black pepper
24 slices crusty French or Italian bread, about ½ inch thick (about ½ ounce per slice)
1   garlic clove, cut in half

ROSEMARY

Rosemary has long been associated with memory, and used as a symbol for remembrance of significant events. During the Middle Ages, brides would wear headpieces made from rosemary to symbolize remembrance of their family, and of their wedding day. Greeks and Romans would throw rosemary sprigs into graves as a symbol of remembrance of the departed.

Garnish
¼   teaspoon Pecorino Romano cheese per slice

1. Preheat the oven to 400°F. Line a baking sheet with parchment paper and set aside. Add the cauliflower, thyme, and rosemary to a pot of boiling water. Boil for about 10 minutes, until the cauliflower is tender. Drain. Discard the thyme and rosemary sprigs.

2. Transfer the cauliflower to a bowl. Mix in the olive oil, lemon juice, parsley, Garlic & Herb seasoning, and black pepper. Mash the mixture well with a fork.

3. Place the bread slices on the prepared baking sheet. Toast the bread for about 3 minutes, until lightly toasted. Remove the bread from the oven and immediately rub each piece with the fresh garlic. Spread the cauliflower mixture onto each bread slice. Garnish with Pecorino Romano cheese.

BASIC NUTRITIONAL VALUES

Calories 150
  Calories from Fat 65
Total Fat 7.0 g
  Saturated Fat 1.0 g
  Trans Fat 0 g
Cholesterol 0 mg
Sodium 200 mg
Total Carbohydrate 18 g
  Dietary Fiber 2 g
  Sugars 2 g
Protein 4 g

Tomato Corn Salsa

10 SERVINGS/SERVING SIZE: ½ CUP

PREPARATION TIME: 20 MINUTES

COOK TIME: 10 MINUTES

Don't open a jar of just any old salsa to serve your special guests. Treat them to a homemade tomato corn salsa that goes well with chips, crackers, and hollow vegetables such as celery and endive leaves. The supercrunchy texture serves well as a premeal palate pleaser.

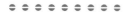

3 large ears fresh corn, peeled and husks removed
2 large tomatoes, cut into ¼-inch dice
⅓ cup peeled and diced jicama
⅓ cup diced red onion
¼ cup chopped fresh cilantro
⅓ cup freshly squeezed lime juice
1 jalapeño pepper, seeded and minced
2 teaspoons salt-free Caribbean Citrus seasoning
1 garlic clove, minced

1. Bring a large pot of water to a boil. Add the corn and cook for 2 to 3 minutes. Turn off the heat and let the corn stand in the water for 5 minutes. Drain and rinse the corn with cold water to stop the cooking. Pat dry with paper towels.

2. Scrape the corn kernels off each cob with a sharp knife into a large bowl. Add the remaining ingredients and mix well. Cover and refrigerate for several hours.

BASIC NUTRITIONAL VALUES

Calories 50
  Calories from Fat 5
Total Fat 0.5 g
  Saturated Fat 0 g
  Trans Fat 0 g
Cholesterol 0 mg
Sodium 0 mg
Total Carbohydrate 11 g
  Dietary Fiber 2 g
  Sugars 3 g
Protein 2 g

Potato Pockets

21 SERVINGS/SERVING SIZE: 1 ROLL, ¼ CUP SAUCE

PREPARATION TIME: 35 MINUTES

COOK TIME: 25 MINUTES

These potato pockets are a variation on deep-fried Indian potato pastries called samosas. These still contain such spices as turmeric, cumin, and cayenne, which are reminiscent of the traditional Indian treat, but can be enjoyed without all the fat.

● ● ● ● ● ● ● ●

BASIC NUTRITIONAL VALUES

Calories 195
  Calories from Fat 25
Total Fat 3.0 g
  Saturated Fat 0 g
  Trans Fat 0 g
Cholesterol 0 mg
Sodium 130 mg
Total Carbohydrate 39 g
  Dietary Fiber 3 g
  Sugars 18 g
Protein 4 g

1 teaspoon olive oil
1 onion, chopped
1 garlic clove, minced
6 medium-size red potatoes, scrubbed, boiled, and diced
1 cup cooked yellow lentils
1 tablespoon ground mustard
1 tablespoon ground turmeric
1 tablespoon ground cumin
1 teaspoon cayenne pepper
¼ cup finely chopped fresh cilantro
Freshly ground pepper
1 (16-ounce) package egg roll wrappers
3 to 4 tablespoons vegetable oil for sautéing

TURMERIC

Turmeric belongs to the same family as ginger, and it resembles ginger in its fresh form. It is commonly used as a colorant in cheese and margarine. In South Asia, a paste of turmeric is thought to improve complexion because of its antioxidant and antibacterial properties. A facial mask is made by mixing 1 teaspoon of ground turmeric, 1 tablespoon of honey, and 3 tablespoons of yogurt. Apply it for 10 minutes, then rinse it off.

1. In a large skillet, heat the 1 teaspoon of olive oil. Sauté the onion and garlic until transparent, about 5 minutes. In a large bowl, mash the potatoes, lentils, onion mixture, spices, and cilantro together. Soak the wonton wrappers individually in a bowl of warm water for 10 seconds.

2. Place a dampened wonton on a cutting board, scoop 1 to 2 tablespoons of the potato mixture onto the wrapper, and pull one corner over the mixture. Fold in two opposite sides, and then roll until the potato mixture is all within the wrapper.

3. In the same skillet, heat 2 tablespoons of the vegetable oil over medium heat. Drop a tiny bit of leftover potato mixture into the oil; it should begin to sizzle immediately. If the oil splashes, turn the temperature down. If it doesn't sizzle, turn up the heat and repeat.

4. Drop each wonton into the heated oil and cook for about 1 minute on each side, or until the wonton is browned and bubbly. When completely cooked, drop the wonton onto a paper towel to catch any excess oil. You may need to replenish the oil with 1 or 2 more tablespoons of oil as you cook the remaining wontons.

5. Serve with Peach Chutney (recipe follows).

Peach Chutney

1 cup apple cider vinegar
1 cup sugar
1 garlic clove, minced
1 cup golden raisins
6 peaches, peeled, pitted, and chopped
1 teaspoon ground cloves

1. Bring the vinegar and sugar to a boil, stirring constantly, until the sugar is completely dissolved and the mixture bubbles. Mix in the garlic, raisins, peaches, and ground cloves. Simmer for 20 minutes.

2. When the peaches appear to be soft, mash with a potato masher. The mixture will become syrupy and sweet and will turn a rich caramel color.

Indian Chicken Skewers

8 SERVINGS/SERVING SIZE: 1 SKEWER

PREPARATION TIME: 20 MINUTES

MARINATING TIME: 30 MINUTES

COOK TIME: 12 MINUTES

I just love Indian Chicken Skewers. To turn this appetizer into a full meal, remove the meat and vegetables from the skewers and stir into cooked brown rice. If you like it spicy, double the chili powder.

❧ ❧ ❧ ❧ ❧ ❧ ❧ ❧ ❧

1	teaspoon chili powder or chipotle chili pepper powder
2	teaspoons garam masala
1	teaspoon garlic powder
1	teaspoon curry powder
1	(1-inch) piece fresh ginger, chopped finely or crushed
⅓	cup plain low-fat or nonfat Greek yogurt
10	ounces boneless, skinless chicken breasts, cut into 1- to 1½-inch pieces (16 pieces in all)
1	small zucchini
1	medium-size red bell pepper
2	medium-size onions
2	teaspoons olive oil

1. Soak eight 8-inch wooden skewers in a pan of hot water for 1 hour.

2. Meanwhile, in a small bowl, mix together the chili powder, garam masala, garlic powder, curry powder, and ginger. This should make almost 3 tablespoons.

3. Divide the spice mixture and mix half (about 1½ tablespoons) into the yogurt with a fork until well blended. In a separate bowl, toss the spiced yogurt with the chicken pieces until well coated. Cover with plastic wrap and refrigerate for 30 minutes.

3. While the chicken is chilling, cut the zucchini in half lengthwise and then cut each half into eight pieces, for a total of sixteen pieces. Cut the red bell pepper into sixteen 1½- to 2-inch pieces and cut each onion into eighths.

4. Toss the vegetables with the rest of the spice mixture in a separate bowl. Set aside.

5. Meanwhile, heat the oven to low-broil. Assemble the skewers by threading each soaked skewer in this order: zucchini, red pepper, onion, chicken, and then repeat.

6. Line sheet pans with aluminum foil and spray with cooking spray. Arrange the skewers on the prepared pans. Bake for 10 to 12 minutes, until the chicken and vegetables are browned.

BASIC NUTRITIONAL VALUES

Calories 80
  Calories from Fat 20
Total Fat 2.5 g
  Saturated Fat 0 g
  Trans Fat 0 g
Cholesterol 20 mg
Sodium 30 mg
Total Carbohydrate 7 g
  Dietary Fiber 2 g
  Sugars 3 g
Protein 9 g

Chimichurri Stuffed Mushrooms

8 SERVINGS/SERVING SIZE: 2 MUSHROOMS

PREPARATION TIME: 20 MINUTES

COOK TIME: 15 MINUTES

These stuffed mushrooms make an elegant appetizer for any occasion. Walnuts finish the dish and add crunch and color. With an abundance of fresh herbs and lemon zest, you won't even miss the salt.

● ● ● ● ● ● ● ● ●

2 (8-ounce) packages whole mushrooms, washed, dried, and stems removed
2 teaspoons olive oil
¼ cup finely chopped onion
2 garlic cloves, minced
1 (10-ounce) package frozen chopped spinach, squeezed dry
½ cup packed, finely chopped fresh parsley
½ cup packed, finely chopped fresh cilantro
2 tablespoons finely chopped fresh oregano, or 2 teaspoons dried
1 tablespoon sherry vinegar
1 tablespoon freshly squeezed lemon juice
1 teaspoon fresh lemon zest
1 tablespoon chopped walnuts

1. Preheat the oven to 425°F. Line a heavy-duty sheet pan with aluminum foil. Finely chop the mushroom stems.

2. In a medium-size sauté pan, heat the oil. Sauté the onions, garlic, and mushroom stems until soft, 5 to 10 minutes over medium heat. Add the spinach, herbs, sherry vinegar, lemon juice, and lemon zest. Mix well.

3. Place the mushroom caps hollow side up on the prepared sheet pan. Mound a spoonful of the spinach mixture in the hollow of each mushroom. (You should use it all.) Sprinkle each mushroom with chopped walnuts.

4. Bake for 15 minutes. Serve.

BASIC NUTRITIONAL VALUES

Calories 45
  Calories from Fat 20
Total Fat 2.0 g
  Saturated Fat 0 g
  Trans Fat 0 g
Cholesterol 0 mg
Sodium 35 mg
Total Carbohydrate 5 g
  Dietary Fiber 2 g
  Sugars 2 g
Protein 3 g

Garlic and Herb Scallops

8 SERVINGS/SERVING SIZE: 2 OUNCES

PREPARATION TIME: 15 MINUTES

COOK TIME: 10 MINUTES

A recipe for perfectly seared scallops is a basic necessity for any home cook. Scallops can be tricky; here I've shown you the proper way to get a good sear on them. The trick is to not overcrowd them in the pan and only sear for about 2 minutes per side. Simply pair them with an easy sauce redolent with garlic and shallots.

❧ ❧ ❧ ❧ ❧ ❧ ❧ ❧

BASIC NUTRITIONAL VALUES

Calories 115
  Calories from Fat 65
Total Fat 7.0 g
  Saturated Fat 2.5 g
  Trans Fat 0 g
Cholesterol 25 mg
Sodium 125 mg
Total Carbohydrate 4 g
  Dietary Fiber 0 g
  Sugars 0 g
Protein 9 g

1 pound large, fresh, dry-packed sea scallops (cut in half any that are too large)
1 tablespoon salt-free Garlic & Herb seasoning
2 tablespoons olive oil
2 tablespoons unsalted butter
½ cup dry white wine
1 large shallot, minced
1 garlic clove, minced finely
½ cup low-sodium, reduced-fat chicken stock (page 123)
2 teaspoons freshly squeezed lemon juice

Garnish
¼ cup minced fresh parsley

1. Coat each scallop on both sides with the Garlic & Herb seasoning.

2. Heat a large, heavy skillet (not nonstick) over medium-high heat. Heat the olive oil and 2 teaspoons of the butter. Sear the scallops on both sides for about 2 minutes per side, or until just cooked through. Cook them in two batches if necessary; do not crowd the pan. Transfer the scallops to a plate and set aside.

3. Add the wine, scraping up any browned bits. Reduce the wine until almost evaporated. Add the shallot and garlic and sauté for 3 to 4 minutes. Add the stock and reduce the volume by half. Swirl in the remaining butter.

4. Add back the scallops and lemon juice and cook for 1 minute. Garnish with minced parsley.

Eggplant Tomato Stacks

5 SERVINGS/SERVING SIZE: 3 STACKS

PREPARATION TIME: 10 MINUTES

COOK TIME: 10 MINUTES

This recipe is a wonderful eggplant appetizer. Summer vegetables deserve really good aged balsamic vinegar—it's thick, sweet, and oh so delicious. Choose tomatoes of various sizes to match the diameter of your eggplant slices. Herbes de Provence really makes these eggplant stacks very special.

＊ ＊ ＊ ＊ ＊ ＊ ＊ ＊ ＊

3 tomatoes, cut into ½-inch slices (about 15 slices)

4 teaspoons olive oil

½ teaspoon herbes de Provence

1 medium-size eggplant with strips of skin removed so that it has long purple and white stripes, cut in ½-inch slices (about 15 slices)

Fresh cracked pepper

3 tablespoons aged balsamic vinegar

2 teaspoons snipped fresh rosemary

1. Preheat the oven to 450°F. Line a jelly-roll pan or cookie sheet with parchment paper. Place the tomato slices on the pan.

2. Brush the top of the tomato slices with 1 tablespoon of the olive oil. Sprinkle with herbes de Provence. Bake for 10 minutes.

3. Meanwhile, lightly brush a grill pan with the remaining 1 teaspoon of olive oil. Preheat the pan over medium-high heat.

4. In batches, cook the eggplant slices for 2 to 3 minutes, or until grill marks appear. Flip and cook for another 1 minute.

5. Transfer the eggplant slices to a serving tray and place one tomato slice on each eggplant slice. Sprinkle with fresh cracked pepper, balsamic vinegar, and rosemary.

BASIC NUTRITIONAL VALUES

Calories 90

  Calories from Fat 35

Total Fat 4.0 g

  Saturated Fat 0.5 g

  Trans Fat 0 g

Cholesterol 0 mg

Sodium 5 mg

Total Carbohydrate 14 g

  Dietary Fiber 4 g

  Sugars 7 g

Protein 2 g

DID YOU KNOW?

Over the past four decades, the average sodium intake in the United States increased 38 percent among adult males and 57 percent among adult females. The culprits? More processed foods and more meals outside the home.

Pasta and Smoked Trout Salad with Cilantro Salsa Verde

6 SERVINGS/SERVING SIZE: ½ CUP

PREPARATION TIME: 20 MINUTES

COOK TIME: 8 MINUTES

When I visited Australia, I was bowled over by the abundance of fresh herbs used in daily cooking. I visited several bustling gardens teeming with home cooks anxious to sniff and feel the hundreds of varieties of beautiful herb plants. This is a favorite dish from Down Under.

❀ ❀ ❀ ❀ ❀ ❀ ❀ ❀ ❀

BASIC NUTRITIONAL VALUES

Calories 325
  Calories from Fat 100
Total Fat 11.0 g
  Saturated Fat 1.5 g
  Trans Fat 0 g
  Polyunsaturated Fat 2.0 g
  Monounsaturated Fat 6.0 g
Cholesterol 40 mg
Sodium 195 mg
Total Carbohydrate 36 g
  Dietary Fiber 5 g
  Sugars 3 g
Protein 22 g

8 ounces small pasta (shells or elbows)
1 cup frozen peas
1 tablespoon olive oil
6 scallions, white part only, sliced thinly
2 tablespoons toasted, slivered almonds
½ teaspoon paprika
Zest and juice of 1 lemon

Cilantro Salsa Verde
2 teaspoons white wine vinegar
2 teaspoons olive oil
½ cup chopped fresh flat-leaf parsley
½ cup stemmed, chopped fresh cilantro
1 garlic clove
1 green chile, seeded and chopped (optional)

8 ounces smoked trout
6 cups mixed greens

1. Cook the pasta according to the package directions, except do not add salt to the water. During the last 2 minutes of cooking, add the frozen peas. Drain the pasta, rinse with cold water, drain again. Set aside.

2. Place the pasta and peas in a large serving bowl. Add the olive oil, scallions, almonds, paprika, lemon zest, and lemon juice.

3. Blend all the Cilantro Salsa Verde ingredients together in a blender or with an immersion blender. Add half of the Cilantro Salsa Verde to the pasta and peas and toss well.

4. Remove the skin from the trout and use a fork to flake the flesh from the bone. Add the trout to the pasta and peas. Cover and refrigerate for several hours. Add the remaining Cilantro Salsa Verde just prior to serving.

5. Divide the salad greens among six serving plates and top each with the Pasta Trout Salad.

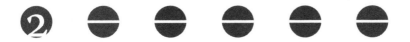

Snacks

Tandoori Snack Mix

MAKES 3 CUPS OR 12 SERVINGS/SERVING SIZE: ¼ CUP

PREPARATION TIME: 5 MINUTES

COOK TIME: 40 MINUTES

Cashews need not be soaked in salt! Their nutty flavor is so much better, sans the sodium, in this fun snack flavored with intriguing tandoori-style seasoning. The sweet dried fruits balance out the slightly peppery taste of the spice.

❀ ❀ ❀ ❀ ❀ ❀ ❀ ❀ ❀

2   cups raw cashews
¼   cup canola oil
½   tablespoon salt-free tandoori-style seasoning
1   cup dried bananas
1   cup golden raisins

1. Preheat the oven to 300°F. Combine the cashews and oil and toss well. Spread out in a single layer on a baking sheet and toast the cashews for about 20 minutes, stirring every 10 minutes. Add the tandoori-style seasoning and dried bananas to the nuts, mix well, and spread out again in an even, single layer.

2. Continue to roast for another 20 minutes, stirring every 10 minutes. Remove the pan from the oven, add the golden raisins, and serve. Store in a covered container.

BASIC NUTRITIONAL VALUES

Calories 235
  Calories from Fat 135
Total Fat 15.0 g
  Saturated Fat 2.0 g
  Trans Fat 0 g
Cholesterol 0 mg
Sodium 0 mg
Total Carbohydrate 24 g
  Dietary Fiber 2 g
  Sugars 13 g
Protein 5 g

Sweet and Spicy Walnuts

MAKES 1 POUND OR 18
  SERVINGS/SERVING SIZE: ¼ CUP

PREPARATION TIME: 5 MINUTES

COOK TIME: 20 MINUTES

These addictive spiced walnuts are great for snacking and for garnishing salads and soups. Why pay for expensive pre-pared nut mixtures when you can make your own for pennies—and keep the sodium out and the flavor in!

❖ ❖ ❖ ❖ ❖ ❖ ❖ ❖ ❖

¼ cup unsalted butter
¾ cup brown sugar
¼ cup water
2 tablespoons salt-free Caribbean Citrus seasoning
1 pound halved walnuts

1. Preheat the oven to 375°F. Line a large baking sheet with parchment paper (if necessary, use two baking sheets).

2. In a large saucepan, melt the butter over medium heat. Add the brown sugar, water, and Caribbean Citrus seasoning and mix well. Bring to a boil and cook for 2 minutes; the mixture will thicken. Stir often to prevent the sugar from burning. Turn off the heat and fold in the walnuts to coat the nuts with the brown sugar mixture.

3. Turn out the walnuts onto the prepared baking sheet(s). Spread the nuts into one layer.

4. Bake the nuts for 12 to 15 minutes—watching the nuts carefully to make sure they don't burn—until they are toasted and feel somewhat dry to the touch. The nuts will still have a bit of runny brown sugar mixture on them. Remove the nuts from the oven and let cool at room temperature. Any loose brown sugar mixture will harden.

5. Store the nuts in a covered container. Keeps for 1 to 2 weeks.

BASIC NUTRITIONAL VALUES

Calories 225
  Calories from Fat 170
Total Fat 19.0 g
  Saturated Fat 3.0 g
  Trans Fat 0 g
Cholesterol 5 mg
Sodium 25 mg
Total Carbohydrate 13 g
  Dietary Fiber 2 g
  Sugars 10 g
Protein 4 g

Guacamole

16 SERVINGS/SERVING SIZE: ¼ CUP

PREPARATION TIME: 15 MINUTES

COOK TIME: 0

I have many colleagues who continue to use salt in their guacamole, but I really can't understand why. With the rich buttery texture of the avocado coupled with fresh lime juice and delightful heat from the Southwest Chipotle seasoning, you'll find that added salt is unnecessary.

4   medium-size ripe avocados
3   tablespoons freshly squeezed lime juice
2   tablespoons salt-free Southwest Chipotle seasoning
1   medium-size tomato, seeded and diced
½   small Vidalia onion, minced
¼   cup minced fresh cilantro
1   serrano chile pepper, seeded and finely minced

1. Pit and peel the avocados. Place the avocado flesh in a large bowl. With a potato masher, mash the avocados coarsely. Mix together the lime juice and Southwest Chipotle seasoning, add to the avocados, and continue to mash until the desired consistency is reached.

2. Fold in the tomato, onion, cilantro, and serrano pepper until well mixed. Cover and refrigerate for 1 hour prior to serving.

BASIC NUTRITIONAL VALUES

Calories 65
   Calories from Fat 55
Total Fat 6.0 g
   Saturated Fat 1.0 g
   Trans Fat 0 g
Cholesterol 0 mg
Sodium 10 mg
Total Carbohydrate 4 g
   Dietary Fiber 3 g
   Sugars 1 g
Protein 1 g

Italian Shrimp and Tomato Bruschetta

8 SERVINGS/SERVING SIZE: 1 BREAD SLICE

PREPARATION TIME: 20 MINUTES

COOK TIME: 15 MINUTES

There are so many variations of bruschetta that I learned to make while in Italy. One of my favorites was tiny shrimp sautéed with ripe tomatoes, Italian seasoning, and drizzles of good balsamic vinegar. The shrimp mixture itself is also great over pasta or rice.

❦ ❦ ❦ ❦ ❦ ❦ ❦ ❦ ❦

BASIC NUTRITIONAL VALUES

Calories 150
  Calories from Fat 65
Total Fat 7.0 g
  Saturated Fat 1.0 g
  Trans Fat 0 g
Cholesterol 15 mg
Sodium 180 mg
Total Carbohydrate 17 g
  Dietary Fiber 1 g
  Sugars 2 g
Protein 5 g

8 slices French or Italian bread, about 1 inch thick (about 1 ounce each)
¼ cup olive oil
2 garlic cloves, mashed to a paste
2 teaspoons salt-free Italian seasoning
½ medium-size onion
½ cup diced grape tomatoes
2 teaspoons balsamic vinegar
1 teaspoon sugar
12 medium-size cooked, peeled, and deveined shrimp, diced
5 large fresh basil leaves, sliced into thin strips

1. Preheat the oven to 375°F. Slice the bread into eight slices on a diagonal. Line a baking sheet with parchment paper. Arrange the bread slices on the baking sheet in one layer.

2. Meanwhile, combine all but 1 tablespoon of the olive oil, the garlic, and the Italian seasoning in a small bowl.

BASIL

With over sixty varieties to choose from, there is a type of basil to complement any dish. Store basil as you would fresh flowers: cut off the ends and place in a vase with room temperature water, and change the water daily. Given proper conditions, the basil stems will develop roots and will keep for weeks. Basil can also be frozen, whole or chopped, in a sealed plastic bag.

3. Brush each slice of bread with the olive oil mixture. Set aside.

4. Heat the remaining 1 tablespoon of olive oil in a large skillet over medium-low heat. Add the onion and sauté for 7 to 8 minutes, until the onion is soft. Add the grape tomatoes and sauté for 2 minutes. Add the balsamic vinegar and sauté until the vinegar evaporates. Add the sugar and cook for 1 minute. Add the shrimp and cook for 1 minute. Add the basil leaves.

5. Bake the bread slices for 3 to 4 minutes, just until lightly toasted. Divide the shrimp mixture evenly among all the bread slices and serve.

Spiced Yogurt Dip

MAKES 2 CUPS OR 16
SERVINGS/SERVING SIZE: 2
TABLESPOONS

PREPARATION TIME: 10 MINUTES

COOK TIME: 0

In this dip, use the whole seeds of coriander and cumin rather than purchasing them already ground. The heady fragrance of toasted seeds, followed by crushing them to release their natural oils, makes this dip very special. Use this to top seared salmon or any grilled lamb dish; it is truly delicious!

❈ ❈ ❈ ❈ ❈ ❈ ❈ ❈ ❈

2   teaspoons coriander seeds
2   teaspoons cumin seeds
1   teaspoon ground turmeric
½   teaspoon chili powder
⅛   teaspoon ground ginger
2   cups plain nonfat Greek yogurt
2 to 3   tablespoons freshly squeezed lime juice
1   teaspoon honey

Garnish
1   tablespoon finely minced red onion or scallion

1. In a small, dry skillet, toast the coriander and cumin seeds until fragrant, about 2 minutes. Transfer the seeds to a coffee or spice grinder and grind to a powder.

2. Place the ground coriander and cumin in a bowl. Add the turmeric, chili powder, and ginger and mix well. Fold in the yogurt, lime juice, and honey and mix well. Cover and refrigerate for 1 hour to blend the flavor.

3. Serve in a bowl and garnish with chopped red onion or scallion.

BASIC NUTRITIONAL VALUES

Calories 20
  Calories from Fat 0
Total Fat 0.0 g
  Saturated Fat 0 g
  Trans Fat 0 g
Cholesterol 0 mg
Sodium 15 mg
Total Carbohydrate 2 g
  Dietary Fiber 0 g
  Sugars 2 g
Protein 3 g

Salsa Fresca

MAKES 2 CUPS/SERVING SIZE: ½ CUP

PREPARATION TIME: 15 MINUTES

COOK TIME: 0

Why purchase jarred salsa that is unnecessarily loaded with salt? All that is needed for great salsa is fresh cilantro, really ripe tomatoes, and a kick from a seasoning blend such as the Southwest Chipotle used here. This salsa is not saucy; heaps of it can be piled onto a tortilla chip for a hearty snack.

● ● ● ● ● ● ● ●

4   large ripe tomatoes, chopped (seeded if desired)
½   medium-size sweet white onion, diced
1   small jalapeño pepper (seeded if desired), minced
10 sprigs fresh cilantro, chopped
1   large garlic clove, minced
    Juice of 1 lime
2   tablespoons olive oil
1   teaspoon salt-free Southwest Chipotle seasoning

1. Combine all the ingredients in a serving bowl. Let the salsa fresca stand at room temperature for about 15 minutes prior to serving, to allow flavors to mingle.

BASIC NUTRITIONAL VALUES

Calories 115
  Calories from Fat 65
Total Fat 7.0 g
  Saturated Fat 1.0 g
  Trans Fat 0 g
Cholesterol 0 mg
Sodium 20 mg
Total Carbohydrate 13 g
  Dietary Fiber 3 g
  Sugars 8 g
Protein 2 g

Chicken Fingers

4 SERVINGS/SERVING SIZE: 5 NUGGETS
(ABOUT 4 OUNCES)

MARINATING TIME: 24 HOURS

PREPARATION TIME: 15 MINUTES

COOK TIME: 10 MINUTES

Ever look at the sodium content of frozen or take-out chicken fingers? Let me spare you the number; it isn't pretty. Make chicken fingers yourself with a clear conscience by using a zippy seasoning as the chief source of satisfaction.

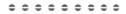

1 pound boneless, skinless chicken breasts
1 cup low-fat buttermilk
1½ cups plain panko bread crumbs
1 tablespoon salt-free Southwest Chipotle seasoning
Freshly ground black pepper
1 tablespoon olive oil

1. Place the chicken in a large plastic bag. With a rolling pin or meat mallet, pound each chicken breast one at a time until thin. Cut all the chicken into a total of twenty pieces. Put the chicken in a large resealable plastic bag and add the buttermilk. Seal the bag and marinate the chicken in the refrigerator overnight.

2. The next day, preheat the oven to 400°F. Line a baking sheet with aluminum foil coated with cooking spray, or with parchment paper. On a plate, combine the panko bread crumbs with the Southwest Chipotle seasoning and pepper to taste. Shake the excess buttermilk off each piece of chicken and roll the chicken in the bread crumb mixture, coating well. Discard any excess panko crumbs.

3. Place the nuggets in a single layer on the prepared baking sheet and drizzle the chicken nuggets with olive oil.

4. Bake the chicken for about 10 minutes, until golden brown.

BASIC NUTRITIONAL VALUES

Calories 215
    Calories from Fat 65
Total Fat 7.0 g
    Saturated Fat 1.5 g
    Trans Fat 0 g
Cholesterol 65 mg
Sodium 110 mg
Total Carbohydrate 11 g
    Dietary Fiber 0 g
    Sugars 2 g
Protein 26 g

Tuscan White Bean Dip

20 SERVINGS/SERVING SIZE: 2
   TABLESPOONS

PREPARATION TIME: 5 MINUTES

CHILLING TIME: 1 TO 2 HOURS

COOK TIME: 0

Bean dips are typically healthy, but can be high in sodium. No need to add salt when you've got intense sun-dried tomatoes, Garlic & Herb seasoning, and fresh lemon in this creamy and very satisfying dip. Use it as a sandwich spread, too!

❧ ❧ ❧ ❧ ❧ ❧ ❧ ❧

1 (15-ounce) can no-salt-added cannellini beans, drained and rinsed
1 (3-ounce) package low-fat cream cheese
2 tablespoons minced rehydrated sun-dried tomatoes (not packed in oil)
2 tablespoons freshly squeezed lemon juice
1 to 2 tablespoons olive oil
1 tablespoon salt-free Garlic & Herb seasoning
1 tablespoon freshly grated Parmesan cheese
Pinch of red pepper flakes
Freshly ground black pepper
3 tablespoons minced scallion (white part only)

1. Combine all the ingredients, except for the scallions, in a food processor or blender and blend until smooth. Add some water if necessary to produce a smooth but thick dip. Taste and correct the seasoning, adding additional lemon juice if desired.

2. Transfer the mixture to a bowl and fold in the scallions. Cover and refrigerate for 1 to 2 hours prior to serving. Serve with pita bread wedges or crudités.

BASIC NUTRITIONAL VALUES

Calories 40
   Calories from Fat 20
Total Fat 2.0 g
   Saturated Fat 0.5 g
   Trans Fat 0 g
Cholesterol 5 mg
Sodium 25 mg
Total Carbohydrate 4 g
   Dietary Fiber 1 g
   Sugars 1 g
Protein 2 g

Garlic and Herb Pita Chips

8 SERVINGS/SERVING SIZE: 4 CHIPS

PREPARATION TIME: 10 MINUTES

COOK TIME: 10 TO 20 MINUTES
(DEPENDING ON THICKNESS OF BREAD)

Traditional pita chips can be doused with salt! Here the subtle flavors of garlic and herbs coat each little wedge. Use these to scoop up your favorite dip or on the side of a hot bowl of soup or chili. These are great with the recipe for Cacik (page 49)

❀ ❀ ❀ ❀ ❀ ❀ ❀ ❀

4 (6-inch) whole wheat pita breads
3 tablespoons olive oil
1½ tablespoons salt-free Garlic & Herb seasoning

1. Preheat the oven to 350°F.

2. Cut each pita into eight wedges. Arrange the wedges in a single layer on a large baking sheet.

3. Combine the oil and 1 tablespoon of the Garlic & Herb seasoning. Brush the mixture over each wedge. Dust the wedges with the remaining ½ tablespoon of the Garlic & Herb Seasoning.

4. Bake the wedges for 10 to 20 minutes, or until crispy.

BASIC NUTRITIONAL VALUES

Calories 120
  Calories from Fat 55
Total Fat 6.0 g
  Saturated Fat 1.0 g
  Trans Fat 0 g
Cholesterol 0 mg
Sodium 150 mg
Total Carbohydrate 16 g
  Dietary Fiber 2 g
  Sugars 0 g
Protein 3 g

Chipotle Chips

3 SERVINGS/SERVING SIZE: 8 CHIPS

PREPARATION TIME: 5 MINUTES

COOK TIME: 20 TO 25 MINUTES

These chips are a healthy alternative to traditional tortilla chips. The zest of lime is a nice balance for the subtle kick of the Southwest Chipotle seasoning.

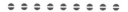

6   (6-inch) corn tortillas
    Olive oil cooking spray
1   tablespoon freshly squeezed lime juice
1   teaspoon salt-free Southwest Chipotle seasoning

1. Preheat the oven to 375°F.

2. Coat both sides of each tortilla with the cooking spray. Cut the tortillas into quarters. Place the tortilla wedges in a single layer on a large baking sheet.

3. Combine the lime juice and Southwest Chipotle seasoning. Brush the mixture on each tortilla wedge.

4. Bake the tortillas for about 20 minutes or until golden and crisp.

BASIC NUTRITIONAL VALUES

Calories 105
  Calories from Fat 15
Total Fat 1.5 g
  Saturated Fat 0 g
  Trans Fat 0 g
Cholesterol 0 mg
Sodium 25 mg
Total Carbohydrate 22 g
  Dietary Fiber 3 g
  Sugars 1 g
Protein 3 g

Creamy Spinach Dip

10 SERVINGS/SERVING SIZE: 2 TABLESPOONS

PREPARATION TIME: 15 MINUTES

COOK TIME: 25 MINUTES (OPTIONAL)

In the '60s, spinach dip was the ubiquitous dip served at every gathering. All you needed to do was to take some spinach and sour cream and dump in that dry and dreadfully high in sodium onion soup mix. I'm glad it's a new century and there are far better ways to prepare this party favorite. The lemon flavoring, achieved with Lemon Pepper seasoning and freshly squeezed lemon juice, really perks up this creamy dip. And by using a combination of low-fat dairy products, you can also feel a whole lot less guilty about snacking on this flavorful treat.

❁ ❁ ❁ ❁ ❁ ❁ ❁ ❁ ❁

½ cup reduced-fat cream cheese
8 ounces plain nonfat Greek yogurt
¼ cup 1% cottage cheese
2 tablespoons low-fat mayonnaise
1 small shallot, minced finely
1 tablespoon freshly squeezed lemon juice
1 teaspoon salt-free Lemon Pepper seasoning
1 (10-ounce) package frozen chopped spinach, thawed, drained, and squeezed dry
2 tablespoons minced fresh chives

1. In a bowl, combine the cream cheese, yogurt, cottage cheese, and mayonnaise and mix until well blended. Add the shallot, lemon juice, and Lemon Pepper seasoning. Mix well.

2. Fold in the spinach and chives and mix well.

To serve this dip warm: Mix as instructed, place in a shallow baking dish, and bake at 350°F for about 25 minutes, or until the dip is hot.

DID YOU KNOW?

"Reduced sodium" on a nutrition label simply means the product is lower in sodium than the regular version; not that it is low in sodium. Always read nutrition labels.

BASIC NUTRITIONAL VALUES

Calories 60
  Calories from Fat 25
Total Fat 3.0 g
  Saturated Fat 1.5 g
  Trans Fat 0 g
Cholesterol 10 mg
Sodium 130 mg
Total Carbohydrate 4 g
  Dietary Fiber 1 g
  Sugars 2 g
Protein 5 g

Cacik

6 SERVINGS/SERVING SIZE: ¼ CUP

PREPARATION TIME: 10 MINUTES

COOK TIME: 0

You may be more familiar with its Greek name, *tzatziki*, but the Turkish dip *cacik* is equally as delicious (and maybe easier to pronounce!). It's one of my very favorite ways to highlight fresh mint. I serve this with grilled lamb and another of my favorites is scooping mounds of it on toasted pita bread.

❂ ❂ ❂ ❂ ❂ ❂ ❂ ❂ ❂

1 tablespoon olive oil
1 teaspoon red wine vinegar
1 garlic clove, minced to a paste
1 cup plain fat-free Greek yogurt
1 (4-inch) piece of cucumber, peeled and grated
2 tablespoons finely chopped fresh mint

Garnish
Mint leaves

1. In a bowl, whisk together the olive oil, vinegar, and garlic. Add the yogurt and mix well.

2. Fold in the cucumber and mint. Cover and refrigerate for several hours. Garnish the bowl with fresh mint leaves. Serve with warmed pita bread.

BASIC NUTRITIONAL VALUES

Calories 70
  Calories from Fat 25
Total Fat 3.0 g
  Saturated Fat 0.5 g
  Trans Fat 0 g
Cholesterol 0 mg
Sodium 45 mg
Total Carbohydrate 5 g
  Dietary Fiber 0 g
  Sugars 5 g
Protein 6 g

Spiced Mango Shake

2 SERVINGS/SERVING SIZE: 1½ CUPS

PREPARATION: 10 MINUTES

COOK TIME: 0

My dear friend Chef Danielle Turner created this refreshing shake that will really wake up the taste buds. And while sodium is not typically an issue with smoothies, this recipe offers a great way to get your palate trained to enjoy a variety of spices in place of sodium in your diet.

❂ ❂ ❂ ❂ ❂ ❂ ❂ ❂ ❂

1½ cups plain fat-free Greek yogurt
 2 cups cubed, ripe mango
 ¼ cup fat-free milk
 ¼ teaspoon ground coriander
 ¼ teaspoon ground ginger

1. Combine all the ingredients in a blender and blend until smooth. Chill thoroughly or serve over ice.

BASIC NUTRITIONAL VALUES

Calories 215
  Calories from Fat 0
Total Fat 0.0 g
  Saturated Fat 0 g
  Trans Fat 0 g
Cholesterol 0 mg
Sodium 85 mg
Total Carbohydrate 37 g
  Dietary Fiber 3 g
  Sugars 33 g
Protein 18 g

Grilled Spiced Peaches

4 SERVINGS/SERVING SIZE: ½ PEACH

PREPARATION TIME: 5 MINUTES

COOK TIME: 6 MINUTES

Instead of having a plain piece of fruit, try these grilled peaches instead. They look fancy; however, they are absolutely simple and delicious. They're perfect for an afternoon pick-me-up or as a special treat for guests. If you want to add some protein to this snack, top your grilled peach half with nonfat Greek yogurt and drizzle with the remaining honey mixture.

✦ ✦ ✦ ✦ ✦ ✦ ✦ ✦ ✦

2 tablespoons honey
2 tablespoons orange juice
½ teaspoon ground cardamom
2 medium-ripe peaches

Garnish
2 to 3 fresh mint leaves, chopped (optional)

1. In a medium-size bowl, whisk together the honey, orange juice, and cardamom and set aside.

2. Cut the peaches along the seam and twist. Use a spoon or a small knife to remove the pit if it clings to the fruit.

3. Toss the peach halves into the honey mixture until well coated.

4. Grill the peach halves cut side down over direct heat for 2 to 3 minutes, or until browned. Flip and cook for an additional 1 to 3 minutes, until they reach desired tenderness. Transfer to a serving platter and sprinkle with chopped mint if desired.

BASIC NUTRITIONAL VALUES

Calories 65
  Calories from Fat 0
Total Fat 0.0 g
  Saturated Fat 0 g
  Trans Fat 0 g
Cholesterol 0 mg
Sodium 0 mg
Total Carbohydrate 17 g
  Dietary Fiber 1 g
  Sugars 15 g
Protein 1 g

Popcorn!

3 SERVINGS/SERVING SIZE: 3 CUPS

PREPARATION TIME: 5 TO 10 MINUTES

If there is one snack food that is drowning in salt, it has to be popcorn. I've always felt that salt actually ruins the nutty flavor of popcorn and that all it really needs is a nice blend of seasonings to enhance its already great taste. So forget about the sodium (and the butter, too!) and enjoy movie-watching with pizza- or curry-flavored popcorn.

❖ ❖ ❖ ❖ ❖ ❖ ❖ ❖ ❖

Pizza-Flavored Popcorn

2 tablespoons freshly grated Parmesan cheese
1 teaspoon garlic powder
1 teaspoon salt-free Italian seasoning
1 teaspoon paprika

Curry-Flavored Popcorn

1 tablespoon curry powder
2 teaspoons sugar
1 teaspoon ground turmeric
 Pinch of cayenne pepper

½ cup unpopped popcorn
1 tablespoon olive oil
 Olive oil or butter-flavored cooking spray

1. For each of the flavored popcorns, combine the seasoning ingredients in a bowl and set aside.

2. Air pop the corn to yield about 3 quarts popcorn. Alternatively, pour 1 tablespoon of olive oil into a large pot and place two kernels of popcorn in it. Turn the heat to medium-high. When the kernels in the pot start to pop, add the rest of the popcorn and cover. Shake the pot several times to ensure even cooking.

3. Transfer the popcorn to a large bowl. Lightly spray the popcorn with cooking oil. Sprinkle on the seasoning of choice and toss gently. The seasonings will last for one year in a covered container.

BASIC NUTRITIONAL VALUES (PIZZA-FLAVORED)

Calories 125 (85 without oil)
 Calories from Fat 65
 (20 without oil)
Total Fat 7.0 g
 (2.0g without oil)
 Saturated Fat 1.5 g
 (1.0 g without oil)
 Trans Fat 0 g
Cholesterol 5 mg
Sodium 30 mg
Total Carbohydrate 14 g
 Dietary Fiber 3 g
 Sugars 1 g
Protein 4 g

BASIC NUTRITIONAL VALUES (CURRY-FLAVORED)

Calories 120 (80 without oil)
 Calories from Fat 55
 (10 without oil)
Total Fat 6.0 g
 (1.0 g without oil)
 Saturated Fat 1.0 g
 (0 g without oil)
 Trans Fat 0 g
Cholesterol 0 mg
Sodium 0 mg
Total Carbohydrate 17 g
 Dietary Fiber 3 g
 Sugars 3 g
Protein 2 g

Champagne Mango Salsa

MAKES 2 CUPS/SERVING SIZE: ¼ CUP

PREPARATION TIME: 20 MINUTES

COOK TIME: 0

A sweet and spicy topping for grilled meats or delicious on its own as a great snack, this salsa gets its flavor from fresh ginger, red onion, and cilantro.

● ● ● ● ● ● ● ● ●

4 ripe Champagne mangoes, chopped finely
3 tablespoons finely minced fresh ginger
⅓ cup finely minced red onion
1 tablespoon minced garlic
1 tablespoon ground cumin
1 teaspoon ground coriander
1 teaspoon cayenne pepper
Freshly ground black pepper
¼ cup chopped fresh cilantro

1. Place the diced mangoes in a medium-size bowl. The consistency of the mangoes should be that of a chunky applesauce.

2. Mix in the ginger and red onion. Add the garlic, cumin, coriander, cayenne, and pepper. Toss in the cilantro.

Note: Champagne mangoes are smaller, sweeter yellow cousins of the mangoes typically found at grocery stores. If you choose to use regular mangoes instead, only use three.

CUMIN

In medieval Europe, it was believed that cumin reinforced fidelity between lovers. Seeds were sprinkled under the bed to promote fidelity. In terms of flavor, black cumin seeds have a sweeter smell and mellower flavor profile. Cumin seeds are best when toasted before grinding.

BASIC NUTRITIONAL VALUES

Calories 60
  Calories from Fat 0
Total Fat 0.0 g
  Saturated Fat 0 g
  Trans Fat 0 g
Cholesterol 0 mg
Sodium 0 mg
Total Carbohydrate 15 g
  Dietary Fiber 2 g
  Sugars 12 g
Protein 1 g

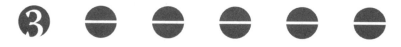

Marinades

Bottled marinades can be dreadfully high in sodium. These homemade ones take no time to prepare and taste so much better than the commercially prepared. So cut the salt and keep the flavor! These indispensable marinades pack a punch of flavor, from the tangy, peppery Herb Marinade to the deeply rich Port Wine Chinese Five-Spice Marinade, I'm sure you'll find endless uses for all of them.

These marinades are made by adding all their ingredients to a food processor or blender and pureeing until combined. Store the marinades in a covered container in the refrigerator for 3 to 4 days. The serving size is 2 tablespoons, based on marinade absorption into an individual portion of seafood, beef, chicken, pork, or lamb.

HOW TO MARINATE

- Marinate seafood for only 30 minutes to 2 hours. Meat and poultry may be marinated for 30 minutes or up to 24 hours for chicken and up to 48 hours for beef, pork, and lamb.
- Marinate all food in a nonreactive container. Stainless-steel bowls, glass, or large plastic resealable bags are best. Cover all food tightly and marinate in the refrigerator for the desired amount of time.

- Remove the food from the refrigerator 15 minutes prior to cooking so the food can come to room temperature; this will ensure even cooking. Remove the food from the marinade, allowing the excess to drip back into the container. Discard the excess marinade. If a plastic bag was used to marinate, do not reuse the bag.

Marinades for Seafood

ITALIAN MARINADE

MAKES 1 CUP OR 8 SERVINGS/SERVING SIZE: 2 TABLESPOONS

PREPARATION TIME: 5 MINUTES

½ cup olive oil
½ cup dry white wine
2 tablespoons minced onion
1 tablespoon salt-free Italian seasoning
1 garlic clove, minced
¼ teaspoon crushed red chili flakes

Combine all the ingredients in a food processor or blender. Store the marinade in a covered container for up to 3 to 4 days.

BASIC NUTRITIONAL VALUES

Calories 135
 Calories from Fat 125
Total Fat 14.0 g
 Saturated Fat 2.0 g
 Trans Fat 0 g
Cholesterol 0 mg
Sodium 0 mg
Total Carbohydrate 1 g
 Dietary Fiber 0 g
 Sugars 0 g
Protein 0 g

LEMON PEPPER MARINADE

MAKES 1 CUP OR 8 SERVINGS/SERVING SIZE: 2 TABLESPOONS

PREPARATION TIME: 5 MINUTES

⅔ cup unsweetened pineapple juice
3 tablespoons brown sugar or honey
3 tablespoons red wine vinegar
2 tablespoons olive oil
1 teaspoon minced crystallized ginger
¼ teaspoon cayenne pepper

Combine all the ingredients in a food processor or blender. Store the marinade in a covered container for up to 3 to 4 days.

BASIC NUTRITIONAL VALUES

Calories 65
 Calories from Fat 30
Total Fat 3.5 g
 Saturated Fat 0 g
 Trans Fat 0 g
Cholesterol 0 mg
Sodium 0 mg
Total Carbohydrate 8 g
 Dietary Fiber 0 g
 Sugars 7 g
Protein 0 g

TROPICAL MARINADE

MAKES 1 CUP OR 8 SERVINGS/SERVING SIZE: 2 TABLESPOONS

PREPARATION TIME: 5 MINUTES

½ cup olive oil
⅓ cup dry white wine
3 tablespoons freshly squeezed lemon juice
1 tablespoon grated fresh lemon zest
2 teaspoons salt-free Lemon Pepper seasoning
1 garlic clove, crushed

Combine all the ingredients in a food processor or blender. Store the marinade in a covered container for up to 3 to 4 days.

BASIC NUTRITIONAL VALUES

Calories 130
 Calories from Fat 125
Total Fat 14.0 g
 Saturated Fat 2.0 g
 Trans Fat 0 g
Cholesterol 0 mg
Sodium 0 mg
Total Carbohydrate 1 g
 Dietary Fiber 0 g
 Sugars 0 g
Protein 0 g

Marinades for Chicken, Beef, Pork, and Lamb

SOUTHWESTERN MARINADE

MAKES 1 CUP OR 8 SERVINGS/SERVING SIZE: 2 TABLESPOONS

PREPARATION TIME: 5 MINUTES

½ cup olive oil

⅓ cup freshly squeezed lime juice

1 tablespoon salt-free Southwest Chipotle seasoning

2 tablespoons minced scallion (white part only)

1 garlic clove, minced

Combine all the ingredients in a food processor or blender. Store the marinade in a covered container for up to 3 to 4 days.

BASIC NUTRITIONAL VALUES

Calories 125
  Calories from Fat 125
Total Fat 14.0 g
  Saturated Fat 2.0 g
  Trans Fat 0 g
Cholesterol 0 mg
Sodium 5 mg
Total Carbohydrate 1 g
  Dietary Fiber 0 g
  Sugars 0 g
Protein 0 g

PORT WINE CHINESE FIVE-SPICE MARINADE

MAKES ¾ CUP OR 6 SERVINGS/SERVING SIZE: 2 TABLESPOONS

PREPARATION TIME: 5 MINUTES

½ cup port wine

¼ cup canola oil

1 tablespoon red wine vinegar

2 teaspoons fresh orange zest

1 teaspoon Chinese five-spice powder

Combine all the ingredients in a food processor or blender. Store the marinade in a covered container for up to 3 to 4 days.

BASIC NUTRITIONAL VALUES

Calories 115
  Calories from Fat 80
Total Fat 9.0 g
  Saturated Fat 0.5 g
  Trans Fat 0 g
Cholesterol 0 mg
Sodium 0 mg
Total Carbohydrate 3 g
  Dietary Fiber 0 g
  Sugars 2 g
Protein 0 g

HERB MARINADE

MAKES 1 CUP OR 8 SERVINGS/SERVING
SIZE: 2 TABLESPOONS

PREPARATION TIME: 5 MINUTES

½ cup olive oil
¼ cup dry red wine
2 tablespoons freshly squeezed lemon juice
2 tablespoons salt-free all-purpose seasoning
1 garlic clove, crushed

Combine all the ingredients in a food processor or blender. Store the marinade in a covered container for up to 3 to 4 days.

BASIC NUTRITIONAL VALUES

Calories 130
  Calories from Fat 125
Total Fat 14.0 g
  Saturated Fat 2.0 g
  Trans Fat 0 g
Cholesterol 0 mg
Sodium 0 mg
Total Carbohydrate 2 g
  Dietary Fiber 0 g
  Sugars 1 g
Protein 0 g

MINT MARINADE

MAKES 1 CUP OR 8 SERVINGS/SERVING
SIZE: 2 TABLESPOONS

PREPARATION TIME: 5 MINUTES

½ cup olive oil
½ cup minced fresh mint
3 tablespoons freshly squeezed lime juice
2 tablespoons white wine vinegar
1 teaspoon Dijon mustard
  Freshly ground black pepper

Combine all the ingredients in a food processor or blender, adding the freshly ground black pepper to taste. Store the marinade in a covered container for up to 3 to 4 days.

BASIC NUTRITIONAL VALUES

Calories 125
  Calories from Fat 125
Total Fat 14.0 g
  Saturated Fat 2.0 g
  Trans Fat 0 g
Cholesterol 0 mg
Sodium 20 mg
Total Carbohydrate 1 g
  Dietary Fiber 0 g
  Sugars 0 g
Protein 0 g

MINT

Peppermint and spearmint are the two most popular mint varieties because of their strong aroma. Peppermint has a high concentration of menthol, which we associate with that lingering fresh minty taste. Menthol is not present in spearmint. So if you want to freshen up your breath, choose to chew a sprig of peppermint!

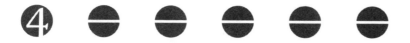

Main Dishes

Caribbean-Style Pork Tenderloin with Melon Salsa

6 SERVINGS/SERVING SIZE: 3 TO 4
OUNCES, ½ CUP SALSA

PREPARATION TIME: 15 MINUTES

MARINATING TIME: 3 HOURS

COOK TIME: 35 MINUTES

Because pork tenderloin is so lean, it takes the right recipe to make it moist. By marinating the pork, then applying a spicy rub, all the juices are sealed in. Adding a side of colorful and healthy salsa turns the humble tenderloin into something special enough to serve guests. Serve the pork cold and sliced in a whole wheat pita bread with the salsa as a relish.

❍ ❍ ❍ ❍ ❍ ❍ ❍ ❍ ❍

BASIC NUTRITIONAL VALUES

Calories 205
 Calories from Fat 40
Total Fat 4.5 g
 Saturated Fat 1.5 g
 Trans Fat 0 g
 Cholesterol 80 mg
Sodium 70 mg
Total Carbohydrate 12 g
 Dietary Fiber 2 g
 Sugars 8 g
 Protein 31 g

2 pork tenderloins (1 pound each), trimmed of excess fat
½ cup freshly squeezed lime juice
2 garlic cloves, minced finely
2 serrano peppers, minced (seeds removed if you like less spicy)
2 tablespoons salt-free Caribbean Citrus seasoning

Melon Salsa
1 large cucumber
1 small cantaloupe, seeded and cut into 1-inch cubes
½ pint cherry tomatoes, halved
2 tablespoons thinly sliced fresh basil
2 tablespoons freshly squeezed lime juice
1 teaspoon sugar

1. Place the pork tenderloins in a large baking dish. Combine the lime juice, garlic, and serrano peppers. Pour over the pork, cover, and refrigerate for 2 to 3 hours.

2. Remove the pork from the marinade and pat the excess marinade from the pork. Rub each tenderloin with the Caribbean Citrus seasoning. Let the pork stand for 10 minutes at room temperature.

3. Heat a gas grill to medium-high or an oven broiler with the rack set 6 inches from the heat source. Grill or broil the pork for 18 to 20 minutes (internal temperature of 150°F).

4. Meanwhile, combine all the salsa ingredients. Set aside.

5. Transfer the pork to a platter and cover with tented foil. Let the pork rest for about 10 minutes. Slice the pork and serve with the salsa on the side.

> **DID YOU KNOW?**
> A 3-ounce broiled pork chop provides 46 milligrams of sodium, whereas 3 ounces of deli ham can contain as much as 1,110 milligrams of sodium.

Italian Chicken with White Beans

4 SERVINGS/SERVING SIZE: 4 OUNCES

PREPARATION TIME: 15 MINUTES

COOK TIME: 1 HOUR

A great, hearty dish for a cold, wintry day. When developing this recipe, I recalled visiting one of my favorite tavernas on a cool day in Florence, Italy, years ago. The chef prepared a special dish that day: a wonderful mélange of tender chicken with white beans in a sauce flavored with the chef's own rich balsamic vinegar. A wonderful food memory is re-created here for your dining pleasure.

⚬ ⚬ ⚬ ⚬ ⚬ ⚬ ⚬ ⚬ ⚬

BASIC NUTRITIONAL VALUES

Calories 335
  Calories from Fat 125
Total Fat 14.0 g
  Saturated Fat 3.0 g
  Trans Fat 0 g
Cholesterol 55 mg
Sodium 75 mg
Total Carbohydrate 31 g
  Dietary Fiber 8 g
  Sugars 9 g
Protein 23 g

1 pound skinless bone-in chicken thighs
   Freshly ground black pepper
2 tablespoons olive oil
⅓ cup dry red wine
1 large onion, diced
3 garlic cloves, minced
2 teaspoons no-salt Italian seasoning
1 (28-ounce) can no-salt-added, whole tomatoes
2 teaspoons good-quality balsamic vinegar
1 (15.5-ounce) can no-salt-added white beans (chickpeas or cannellini beans), drained and rinsed

Garnish
¼ cup sliced fresh basil

1. Sprinkle both sides of the chicken thighs lightly with black pepper. Heat the olive oil in a large skillet or Dutch oven over medium-high heat. Add the chicken thighs, in batches if necessary to avoid crowding the pan. Sear the chicken for 5 to 6 minutes per side. Cover, lower the heat to medium, and cook until the chicken is almost cooked through. Remove the chicken from the pan and set aside.

2. Add the wine, scraping up any browned bits. Add the onion and sauté on medium-low heat for about 10 minutes. Add the garlic and continue to sauté for about 3 minutes. Add the Italian seasoning and sauté for 1 minute.

3. Place the whole tomatoes in a large bowl. With your hands, crush the tomatoes into small pieces, but still leave them a little chunky. Add the tomatoes and their juices to the pan and bring to a boil. Lower the heat and cook over medium heat for 15 to 20 minutes. Add the balsamic vinegar and continue to cook until the sauce is thickened. Add the white beans and cook for 2 minutes, until the beans are heated through.

4. Add back the chicken pieces, nestling them in the sauce. Cook for about 5 minutes, until the chicken is completely cooked through. Garnish with sliced fresh basil.

Cod with Orange

4 SERVINGS/SERVING SIZE: 4 OUNCES

PREPARATION TIME: 10 MINUTES

COOK TIME: 18 MINUTES

There are times you want the lightest food possible. Feel nice and virtuous when you sample this light-as-a-feather cod dish. Simple citrus juices with a high-temperature roast make this dish flavorful and oh so unfussy!

⊜ ⊜ ⊜ ⊜ ⊜ ⊜ ⊜ ⊜

1   pound cod fillets
3   large, juicy oranges
½   lime
1   tablespoon fresh orange zest
2   tablespoons olive oil
2   teaspoons salt-free all-purpose seasoning
3   tablespoons toasted pine nuts

1. Arrange the cod in a baking dish. Squeeze two of the oranges and the lime over the fish. Add the orange zest, olive oil, and all-purpose seasoning. Turn the fish over to completely coat both sides. Cover the fish and marinate for 2 hours, occasionally spooning the marinade over the fish.

2. Preheat the oven to 400°F. Slice the remaining orange into thin slices. Place the slices on the fish. Roast the fish for 15 minutes, or until it is cooked through and no longer translucent.

3. Baste the fish with the marinade, sprinkle it with pine nuts, and return it to the oven for 3 to 4 minutes.

4. Serve the cod with the pan juices.

BASIC NUTRITIONAL VALUES

Calories 265
    Calories from Fat 110
Total Fat 12.0 g
    Saturated Fat 1.5 g
    Trans Fat 0 g
Cholesterol 50 mg
Sodium 70 mg
Total Carbohydrate 18 g
    Dietary Fiber 4 g
    Sugars 13 g
Protein 23 g

Asian-Style Meat Loaf

6 SERVINGS/SERVING SIZE: 4 OUNCES

PREPARATION TIME: 15 MINUTES

COOK TIME: 30 MINUTES

Meat loaf can be awfully high in sodium, but not here. I've eliminated the usual tomato sauce topping in favor of developing the flavor inside the meat loaf. The crunch of the water chestnuts is a fun addition. The all-purpose seasoning blends beautifully throughout the loaf; there is absolutely no reason whatsoever to add sprinkles of salt.

- 2 teaspoons toasted sesame oil
- ½ cup minced onion
- 2 garlic cloves, minced
- 2 teaspoons peeled and grated fresh ginger
- 1 pound lean ground beef (93% lean)
- 2 tablespoons salt-free all-purpose seasoning
- 1 egg, beaten
- ¾ cup plain dry bread crumbs
- ½ cup minced canned water chestnuts
- 3 tablespoons dry sherry

1. Preheat the oven to 350°F. Line a baking sheet with parchment paper.

2. Heat the sesame oil in a skillet over medium heat. Add the onion and sauté for 3 minutes. Add the garlic and ginger and sauté for 2 minutes. Transfer the onion mixture to a large bowl.

3. Add all the remaining ingredients to the onion mixture and mix well.

4. Turn out the meat mixture onto the baking sheet and form it into an oblong loaf shape. Bake the meat loaf for 40 to 50 minutes, until golden brown and crusty. Let the meat loaf stand for 15 minutes prior to slicing.

BASIC NUTRITIONAL VALUES

Calories 210
  Calories from Fat 70
Total Fat 8.0 g
  Saturated Fat 2.5 g
  Trans Fat 0 g
Cholesterol 75 mg
Sodium 160 mg
Total Carbohydrate 15 g
  Dietary Fiber 2 g
  Sugars 2 g
Protein 18 g

Tuscan Chicken Thighs with Roasted Vegetables

4 SERVINGS/SERVING SIZE: 1 THIGH
   PLUS ½ CUP VEGETABLES

MARINATING TIME: 4 HOURS OR UP TO
   24 HOURS

PREPARATION TIME: 5 MINUTES PLUS
   10 MINUTES FOR VEGETABLE
   PREPARATION

COOK TIME: 36 MINUTES

Avoid the habit of automatically adding salt to cooked vegetables. When you treat vegetables right, the combination of the high roasting temperature and the right seasonings will highlight the vegetables' natural sweetness.

☻ ☻ ☻ ☻ ☻ ☻ ☻ ☻

BASIC NUTRITIONAL VALUES

Calories 270
   Calories from Fat 155
Total Fat 17.0 g
   Saturated Fat 3.0 g
   Trans Fat 0 g
Cholesterol 45 mg
Sodium 50 mg
Total Carbohydrate 15 g
   Dietary Fiber 3 g
   Sugars 7 g
Protein 14 g

Chicken
3 tablespoons freshly squeezed lemon juice
2 tablespoons olive oil
3 garlic cloves, minced
1 tablespoon salt-free Italian seasoning
1 pound skinless chicken thighs, bone in

Vegetables
2 medium-size red onions, sliced into wedges
2 red bell peppers, seeded, cored, and cut into 1-inch squares
1 large portobello mushroom, cleaned, stem removed, and sliced into ½-inch pieces
2 tablespoons olive oil
1 tablespoon balsamic vinegar
2 teaspoons salt-free Italian seasoning
   Pinch of kosher salt

1. Prepare the chicken: Mix together the lemon juice, olive oil, garlic, and Italian seasoning in a large bowl. Add the chicken thighs, turn to coat, and marinate in the refrigerator 4 hours or up to overnight.

2. The next day, remove the chicken from the refrigerator and allow it to come to room temperature. Preheat the oven to 400°F. Line a broiler pan with aluminum foil. Coat the foil with cooking spray. Line a baking sheet with parchment paper.

3. Meanwhile, prepare the vegetables: In a large bowl, combine the red onion, red bell pepper, portobello mushroom, olive oil, balsamic vinegar, and Italian seasoning. Spread the vegetables onto the parchment paper–lined baking sheet in a single layer.

4. Drain the chicken from the marinade. Place the chicken thighs on the foil-lined broiler tray.

5. Roast the chicken and vegetables for 25 to 30 minutes, until the chicken is cooked through and the vegetables are tender. Remove the vegetables from the oven. Turn the oven to BROIL. Broil the chicken for 2 to 3 minutes per side. Serve the chicken with the vegetables.

Herbed Chicken Salad with White Beans

8 SERVINGS/SERVING SIZE: 1 CUP

PREPARATION TIME: 20 MINUTES

COOK TIME: 10 TO 12 MINUTES

Why settle for chicken salad that you have to pump up with salt? By using two different types of salt-free seasoning blends, you can create many layers of flavors. Here, a bold, salt-free Grilling Blend seasoning harmonizes with salt-free Garlic & Herb seasoning to create a *wow* chicken salad!

⬥ ⬥ ⬥ ⬥ ⬥ ⬥ ⬥ ⬥

1 pound boneless, skinless chicken breasts
1 tablespoon olive oil
2 tablespoons salt-free Grilling Blend seasoning (for beef or chicken)
1 medium-size red bell pepper, cored, seeded, and diced
1 medium-size yellow bell pepper, cored, seeded, and diced
2 celery stalks, diced
1 large carrot, peeled and diced
10 rehydrated sun-dried tomatoes (not oil packed), sliced into thin strips

Vinaigrette
3 tablespoons olive oil
2 tablespoons freshly squeezed lemon juice
2 teaspoons salt-free Garlic & Herb seasoning
1 teaspoon Dijon mustard

1 (15-ounce) can no-salt-added chickpeas or cannellini beans, drained and rinsed.

Garnish
¼ cup sliced fresh basil

1. Prepare an outdoor grill. Coat the rack with cooking spray. Set the temperature to medium-high. Brush the chicken with the 1 tablespoon of olive oil. Roll the chicken breasts in the Grilling Blend seasoning. Grill the chicken for 5 to 6 minutes per side, or until thoroughly cooked through. Transfer the chicken from the grill to a plate and allow to cool slightly.

2. Combine the red and yellow bell peppers, celery, carrot, and sun-dried tomatoes in a large salad bowl.

3. Whisk together the vinaigrette ingredients in a small bowl and set aside.

4. Cut the chicken into 1-inch cubes and add to the vegetables in the bowl. Add the beans. Pour the vinaigrette over the chicken salad and garnish with fresh basil.

BASIC NUTRITIONAL VALUES

Calories 220
  Calories from Fat 90
Total Fat 10.0 g
  Saturated Fat 1.5 g
  Trans Fat 0 g
Cholesterol 35 mg
Sodium 190 mg
Total Carbohydrate 19 g
  Dietary Fiber 5 g
  Sugars 6 g
Protein 17 g

Chipotle Chicken with Sour Cream Sauce

4 SERVINGS/SERVING SIZE: 4 OUNCES

PREPARATION TIME: 10 MINUTES

COOK TIME: 40 MINUTES

Zesty chipotle-flavored chicken gets a cooling sour cream sauce in this simple weekday meal. Try this dish with lean, boneless pork loin chops as well. If you like, add sliced red peppers to this dish.

❂ ❂ ❂ ❂ ❂ ❂ ❂ ❂

BASIC NUTRITIONAL VALUES

Calories 260
   Calories from Fat 125
Total Fat 14.0 g
   Saturated Fat 5.0 g
   Trans Fat 0 g
Cholesterol 85 mg
Sodium 165 mg
Total Carbohydrate 9 g
   Dietary Fiber 1 g
   Sugars 5 g
Protein 23 g

1 tablespoon olive oil
1 pound boneless, skinless chicken thighs
1 tablespoon salt-free Southwest Chipotle seasoning
1 large onion, chopped
2 garlic cloves, minced
½ cup low-sodium, reduced-fat chicken stock (page 123)
½ cup reduced-fat sour cream

Garnish
¼ cup minced fresh parsley

1. Heat 2 teaspoons of the olive oil in a large skillet over medium-high heat. Sprinkle the chicken with the Southwest Chipotle seasoning. Add the chicken to the pan, in batches if necessary to avoid overcrowding, and sear on both sides for 4 to 5 minutes per side, until golden brown. Transfer the chicken to a plate and set aside.

2. Add the remaining teaspoon of oil to the pan. Add the onion and sauté for about 5 minutes, scraping up any browned bits. Add the garlic and sauté for another 2 minutes. Return the chicken to the pan, add the stock, and reduce and bring to a boil. Cover, turn the heat to low, and simmer the chicken for 10 minutes.

3. Remove the skillet from the heat. Quickly whisk in the sour cream. Put the skillet back on the stove and simmer for 1 minute. Garnish with fresh parsley.

Garlic and Herb Lamb Chops with Browned Onions

4 SERVINGS/SERVING SIZE: 1 CHOP

MARINATING TIME: 1 HOUR OR UP TO 24 HOURS

PREPARATION TIME: 10 MINUTES

COOK TIME: 35 MINUTES

What could be better than lamb chops infused with garlic and herbs, then smothered in caramelized onions? It only sounds complicated and the result looks as if you slaved a bit. The natural sugars in the onions are turned on full strength, so no need for any added sodium.

❀ ❀ ❀ ❀ ❀ ❀ ❀ ❀ ❀

BASIC NUTRITIONAL VALUES

Calories 250
   Calories from Fat 155
Total Fat 17.0 g
   Saturated Fat 3.5 g
   Trans Fat 0 g
Cholesterol 45 mg
Sodium 50 mg
Total Carbohydrate 7 g
   Dietary Fiber 1 g
   Sugars 3 g
Protein 15 g

Marinade

3 tablespoons olive oil
3 tablespoons freshly squeezed lemon juice
1 tablespoon salt-free Garlic & Herb seasoning
1 pound lamb loin chops, trimmed of excess fat

2 teaspoons olive oil
½ cup dry white wine
2 cups thinly sliced onion
1 cup water

Garnish

¼ cup sliced basil or minced fresh parsley

1. In a large bowl, mix together the olive oil, lemon juice, and Garlic & Herb seasoning. Add the lamb chops and turn to coat. Cover and marinate in the refrigerator for at least 1 hour or overnight.

2. Heat the 2 teaspoons of oil in a large skillet. Sear the lamb chops for 3 to 4 minutes per side, until golden brown. Cook the lamb chops for additional time as necessary, to the desired doneness. Remove all the lamb chops from the skillet.

3. Add the white wine and reduce to 3 to 4 tablespoons. Add the onion and sauté over medium heat for 10 to 15 minutes. Add ½ cup of the water and continue to cook the onion until the water is completely absorbed. Add the remaining ½ cup of water and cook until the water is absorbed.

4. Return the lamb chops to the pan and reheat a few minutes, or just serve at room temperature. Serve the lamb chops smothered with the onion and garnished with either basil or parsley.

Lemon Pepper Turkey Burgers

4 SERVINGS/SERVING SIZE: 1 BURGER

PREPARATION TIME: 10 MINUTES

COOK TIME: 14 MINUTES

One of my testers just kept repeating over and over again that these were the juiciest turkey burgers she ever tried. Well, I wish I could lay claim to a miracle, but it's simply a matter of food science. Adding salt to meat drains the meat of its juices, hence its flavor. The salt-free Lemon Pepper seasoning, on the other hand, really makes these turkey burgers pop with taste.

⊜ ⊜ ⊜ ⊜ ⊜ ⊜ ⊜ ⊜

1 pound ground turkey
1 tablespoon salt-free Lemon Pepper seasoning
1 cup panko bread crumbs
1 egg, beaten
¼ cup finely minced onion
2 garlic cloves, minced finely, almost to a paste

1. Combine all the ingredients, handling the meat lightly. Form into four burgers.

2. Prepare an outdoor grill with the rack set 6 inches from the heat source. Coat the rack with cooking spray. Grill the burgers over medium-high heat for 5 to 6 minutes per side, until the turkey is cooked through to an internal temperature of 165°F.

DID YOU KNOW?

Cooking at home will always yield lower sodium values than eating out. Consider that some fast-food individual pizzas contain two day's worth of sodium!

BASIC NUTRITIONAL VALUES

Calories 275
  Calories from Fat 110
Total Fat 12.0 g
  Saturated Fat 3.0 g
  Trans Fat 0 g
Cholesterol 125 mg
Sodium 125 mg
Total Carbohydrate 15 g
  Dietary Fiber 1 g
  Sugars 2 g
Protein 26 g

Indian-Style Skirt Steak with Yogurt Relish

4 SERVINGS/SERVING SIZE: 4 OUNCES

PREPARATION TIME: 10 MINUTES

MARINATING TIME: 2 HOURS

COOK TIME: 6 TO 8 MINUTES (FOR RARE)

Grilling a piece of steak can become monotonous, not to mention its rather plain color. Change the look of the steak altogether by using glorious, yellow-hued, salt-free tandoori-style seasoning. The deep, rich, and inviting look of the seasoning will breathe new life into your basic grilling.

❦ ❦ ❦ ❦ ❦ ❦ ❦ ❦ ❦

BASIC NUTRITIONAL VALUES

Calories 290
  Calories from Fat 145
Total Fat 16.0 g
  Saturated Fat 4.5 g
  Trans Fat 0 g
Cholesterol 75 mg
Sodium 95 mg
Total Carbohydrate 5 g
  Dietary Fiber 1 g
  Sugars 3 g
Protein 30 g

1 pound skirt steak, trimmed of excess fat
1 tablespoon salt-free tandoori-style seasoning
2 tablespoons olive oil

Relish
1 cup plain nonfat Greek yogurt
½ cup peeled, seeded, and chopped cucumber
2 teaspoons salt-free tandoori-style seasoning
¼ cup minced scallions
  Pinch of cayenne pepper

1. Cut the steak crosswise into two pieces. Pat the steak dry and arrange flat in a shallow baking pan. Mix together the tandoori-style seasoning and oil and brush this mixture on all sides of the steak, coating well. Cover with plastic wrap and set aside in the refrigerator to marinate for about 2 hours.

2. Meanwhile, combine all the ingredients for the yogurt relish in a medium-size bowl. Cover and refrigerate until serving time.

3. Remove the steak from the refrigerator and bring to room temperature. Preheat an outdoor grill with the rack set about 6 inches from the heat source. Set the heat to high. Coat the grill rack with cooking spray. Or prepare an oven broiler with the rack set 4 inches from the heat source. Cover a broiler tray with aluminum foil and coat the foil with cooking spray.

4. Add the steak to the grill rack or oven broiler tray and grill or broil for 3 to 4 minutes. Turn the steak over and grill or broil for an additional 3 to 4 minutes for rare steak. Cook for additional time as necessary until the steak reaches the desired doneness.

5. Transfer the steak to a carving board. Let the steak rest for 5 minutes. Slice the steak on a bias into ¼-inch-thick slices. Serve the steak with the yogurt relish.

Tequila Lime Chicken

4 SERVINGS/SERVING SIZE: 4 OUNCES

MARINATING TIME: 4 TO 5 HOURS, OR
UP TO 24 HOURS PREPARATION TIME:
5 MINUTES

COOK TIME: 30 MINUTES

This is one of those wonderful fix-and-forget recipes. In just a few hours, chicken legs are infused with a zesty South of the Border flavor with a kick from the marriage of tequila and Caribbean Citrus seasoning. A very versatile marinade; try this with beef, pork, or lamb as well.

● ● ● ● ● ● ● ● ●

BASIC NUTRITIONAL VALUES

Calories 215
    (175 without skin)
Calories from Fat 115
    (80 without skin)
Total Fat 13.0 g
    (9.0 g without skin)
Saturated Fat 3.0 g
    (2.0 g without skin)
Trans Fat 0 g
Cholesterol 50 mg
    (45 mg without skin)
Sodium 55 mg
    (50 mg without skin)
Total Carbohydrate 6 g
Dietary Fiber 0 g
Sugars 4 g
Protein 15 g
    (13 g without skin)

½ cup tequila
½ cup freshly squeezed lime juice
2 tablespoons olive oil, plus 1 teaspoon for brushing if needed
1 tablespoon salt-free Caribbean Citrus seasoning
1 tablespoon honey
1 teaspoon fresh lime zest
1 pound chicken legs

1. In a large bowl, combine the tequila, lime juice, olive oil, Caribbean Citrus seasoning, honey, and lime zest and mix well. Add the chicken legs, cover, and place in the refrigerator to marinate for 4 to 5 hours or overnight.

2. Preheat an outdoor grill with the rack set about 6 inches from the heat source. Set the heat to medium-high. Coat the grill rack with cooking spray. Or prepare an oven broiler with the rack set 6 inches from the heat source. Cover a broiler tray with aluminum foil and coat the foil with cooking spray.

3. Add the chicken legs and grill or broil for 25 to 30 minutes, until the chicken is cooked through to an internal temperature of 180°F. If the chicken appears dry as it cooks, brush each leg with a little olive oil.

Spicy Chicken Thighs with Smothered Peppers and Onions

4 SERVINGS/SERVING SIZE: 2 PIECES
WITH ½ CUP PEPPERS AND ONIONS

PREPARATION TIME: 10 MINUTES

COOK TIME: 35 MINUTES

This is what I refer to as an everyday pantry dish. Take a look in your pantry and I'll bet you have most of these ingredients on hand right now. The honey and lime finish to this dish provides the perfect complement to the spicy Caribbean Citrus seasoning.

❂ ❂ ❂ ❂ ❂ ❂ ❂ ❂ ❂

BASIC NUTRITIONAL VALUES

Calories 290
  Calories from Fat 145
Total Fat 16.0 g
  Saturated Fat 3.5 g
  Trans Fat 0 g
Cholesterol 70 mg
Sodium 80 mg
Total Carbohydrate 17 g
  Dietary Fiber 3 g
  Sugars 10 g
Protein 22 g

1 pound boneless, skinless chicken thighs
1½ tablespoons salt-free Caribbean Citrus seasoning
2 tablespoons olive oil
1 large Vidalia or other sweet onion, halved and sliced thinly
1 large red bell pepper, cored, seeded, and sliced into thin strips
½ small jalapeño pepper, seeded and minced finely
2 garlic cloves, minced
2 tablespoons freshly squeezed lime juice
1 to 2 teaspoons honey

Garnish
¼ cup minced fresh cilantro

1. Sprinkle the chicken with the Caribbean Citrus seasoning. Heat the olive oil in a large skillet over medium-high heat. Sear the chicken thighs for 4 to 5 minutes per side, until golden brown and cooked through. Turn down the heat at any time if the chicken is browning too quickly. Transfer the chicken to a plate, tent with foil, and set aside.

2. Add the onion to the skillet and sauté over medium heat for 6 to 7 minutes. Add the red bell pepper and sauté for another 5 to 6 minutes, until the pepper is tender. Add the jalapeño pepper and garlic and sauté for 2 minutes. Add back the chicken thighs with its accumulated juices and stir to cover with the peppers and onion. Lower the heat to a simmer and cook for 4 to 5 minutes.

3. Mix together the lime juice and honey and drizzle over the chicken. Garnish with the cilantro.

Salmon with Tomato Pepper Salsa

4 SERVINGS/SERVING SIZE: 5 OUNCES, ¾ CUP SALSA

PREPARATION TIME: 30 MINUTES FOR SALSA TO SET AND 15 MINUTES FOR SALMON

COOK TIME: 10 TO 12 MINUTES

Coating salmon with a simple dry rub of brown sugar and Southwest Chipotle seasoning seals in the juices, making the salmon flaky and tender. By repeating the use of the Southwest Chipotle seasoning in the salsa, you get a double whammy of deep flavor.

● ● ● ● ● ● ● ● ●

BASIC NUTRITIONAL VALUES

Calories 375
  Calories from Fat 200
Total Fat 22.0 g
  Saturated Fat 3.5 g
  Trans Fat 0 g
Cholesterol 100 mg
Sodium 95 mg
Total Carbohydrate 11 g
  Dietary Fiber 2 g
  Sugars 7 g
Protein 33 g

Salsa

2 small red tomatoes, seeded and diced
1 small red bell pepper, cored, seeded, and diced
1 small yellow or green bell pepper, cored, seeded, and diced
¼ cup minced fresh cilantro
2 tablespoons olive oil
3 scallions, minced
1 to 2 tablespoons freshly squeezed lime juice
2 teaspoons salt-free Southwest Chipotle seasoning
1 teaspoon sugar

4 salmon fillets (5 ounces each)
2 teaspoons olive oil
1 tablespoon salt-free Southwest Chipotle seasoning
1 tablespoon brown sugar

1. Combine all the ingredients for the salsa. Let the salsa stand at room temperature for about 30 minutes to allow the flavors to mingle.

2. Meanwhile, preheat the oven to 400°F. Line a baking sheet with parchment paper or cover a broiler tray with aluminum foil. Coat the foil with cooking spray.

3. Brush each salmon fillet lightly with olive oil. Combine the Southwest Chipotle seasoning and brown sugar. Rub each salmon fillet with the seasoning mixture.

4. Bake the salmon for 8 to 9 minutes. Turn the oven to broil and broil the salmon 6 inches from the heat source for an additional 2 to 3 minutes, or until the salmon is cooked to your liking and is golden brown. Serve the salmon with the salsa.

Zesty Oven-Fried Chicken

4 SERVINGS/SERVING SIZE: 5 TO 6 OUNCES

PREPARATION TIME: 10 MINUTES

COOK TIME: 40 MINUTES

How easy is this? Just five ingredients to prepare a chicken dish that everyone will love. I've seen these already prepared at the supermarket for three times the price of what you can cook up from scratch. You can use this crumb coating for white fish, too.

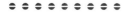

⅓ cup low-fat buttermilk
1 tablespoon salt-free Southwest Chipotle seasoning
1 cup panko bread crumbs
1½ pounds skinless chicken (combination of thighs, drumsticks, and breast), bone in
2 tablespoons olive oil

1. Preheat the oven to 400°F. Line a baking sheet with parchment paper.

2. In a shallow bowl, combine the buttermilk and Southwest Chipotle seasoning. Place the panko bread crumbs on a plate.

> **DID YOU KNOW?**
> From a nutritional standpoint, lowering sodium is only part of the picture. Increasing your intake of potassium and magnesium is just as important for good health. The more processing a food undergoes, the higher its sodium content is and the lesser the potassium it offers.

3. Dip each chicken piece in the buttermilk mixture and roll it in the panko crumbs. Place the chicken on the prepared baking sheet.

4. Drizzle the chicken with olive oil and bake for about 40 minutes, turning once, until the chicken is cooked through and golden brown.

BASIC NUTRITIONAL VALUES

Calories 280
  Calories from Fat 115
Total Fat 13.0 g
  Saturated Fat 2.5 g
  Trans Fat 0 g
Cholesterol 75 mg
Sodium 120 mg
Total Carbohydrate 14 g
  Dietary Fiber 1 g
  Sugars 2 g
Protein 26 g

Sea Bass with Tandoori Spice

4 SERVINGS/SERVING SIZE: 4 OUNCES

MARINATING TIME: 1 HOUR

PREPARATION TIME: 8 MINUTES

COOK TIME: 15 MINUTES

Just a little more exotic than your everyday fish meal, but no more difficult to prepare. After steeping in a cilantro-infused marinade, a light dusting of elegantly colored tandoori-style spice adds a crusty coating to the fish that's at once bold and inviting.

❂ ❂ ❂ ❂ ❂ ❂ ❂ ❂ ❂

BASIC NUTRITIONAL VALUES

Calories 260
  Calories from Fat 125
Total Fat 14.0 g
  Saturated Fat 2.5 g
  Trans Fat 0 g
Cholesterol 60 mg
Sodium 105 mg
Total Carbohydrate 7 g
  Dietary Fiber 2 g
  Sugars 1 g
Protein 27 g

Marinade

3 tablespoons olive oil
¼ cup freshly squeezed lemon juice
1 tablespoon minced fresh cilantro
3 garlic cloves, minced
   Pinch of crushed red pepper

4 sea bass fillets (5 ounces each)
2 tablespoons salt-free tandoori-style seasoning

1. Combine 2 tablespoons of the olive oil with the lemon juice, cilantro, garlic, and crushed red pepper in a baking dish. Add the sea bass fillets and spoon some marinade over the fillets. Cover and refrigerate for 1 hour.

2. Take the baking dish out of the refrigerator and bring to room temperature. Remove the fish from the marinade and reserve the marinade. Rub the fish with the tandoori-style seasoning.

3. Heat the remaining tablespoon of the olive oil in a large, nonstick skillet. Add the fish and cook for 6 to 7 minutes per side, until cooked through and golden brown. Transfer to a platter and keep warm.

4. Pour the marinade into the same skillet. Bring to a boil over medium heat and cook for 1 to 2 minutes, until the sauce is reduced slightly. Drizzle the sauce over the fish and serve.

Apricot Lemon Pepper Chicken

4 SERVINGS/SERVING SIZE: 4 OUNCES

PREPARATION TIME: 15 MINUTES

COOK TIME: 28 MINUTES

Coating this chicken with Lemon Pepper seasoning not only adds taste but creates a delightful, crunchy crust. The sprightly flavor of lemon pepper is further enhanced with sweet apricot preserves and honey. A great go-to dish when you are short on time.

❀ ❀ ❀ ❀ ❀ ❀ ❀ ❀ ❀

1 pound boneless, skinless chicken thighs
1½ tablespoons salt-free Lemon Pepper seasoning
1½ tablespoons canola oil
1 large shallot, sliced thinly
2 tablespoons low-sodium, reduced-fat chicken stock (page 123)
1 large garlic clove, minced
½ cup apricot preserves
1 tablespoon freshly squeezed lemon juice
1 tablespoon honey
1 teaspoon cider vinegar

Garnish
2 tablespoons finely minced fresh parsley

1. Lightly coat both sides of the chicken thighs with the Lemon Pepper seasoning.

2. Heat the oil in a large skillet over medium heat. Add the chicken in two batches, sautéing on both sides for 6 to 7 minutes per side. Transfer the chicken to a plate and set aside.

3. Add the shallots to the pan and sauté over medium-low heat for 6 to 7 minutes. Add the chicken stock and garlic and sauté for 2 to 3 minutes.

4. In a bowl, combine the preserves, lemon juice, honey, and cider vinegar. Add the mixture to the shallots and cook for 1 minute. Return the chicken to the pan and simmer over low heat for 3 minutes. Garnish with chopped parsley and serve.

BASIC NUTRITIONAL VALUES

Calories 345
  Calories from Fat 125
Total Fat 14.0 g
  Saturated Fat 2.5 g
  Trans Fat 0 g
Cholesterol 70 mg
Sodium 100 mg
Total Carbohydrate 35 g
  Dietary Fiber 1 g
  Sugars 24 g
Protein 20 g

Shrimp, Mango, and Kiwi Salad

4 SERVINGS/SERVING SIZE: ¾ CUP

PREPARATION TIME: 25 MINUTES

COOK TIME: 5 MINUTES

The ingredient list may look long, but this dish is long on flavor as well. Actually, it's one of the easiest recipes in this collection and so refreshing on a hot summer day. Use your imagination and try different fruits such as papaya or pineapple in place of the mango and kiwi. Visually, this salad is stunning.

≎ ≎ ≎ ≎ ≎ ≎ ≎ ≎ ≎

BASIC NUTRITIONAL VALUES

Calories 360
  Calories from Fat 200
Total Fat 22.0 g
  Saturated Fat 3.0 g
  Trans Fat 0 g
Cholesterol 130 mg
Sodium 175 mg
Total Carbohydrate 27 g
  Dietary Fiber 4 g
  Sugars 20 g
Protein 16 g

1 pound large shrimp, peeled and deveined
1 tablespoon salt-free Caribbean Citrus seasoning
2 tablespoons canola oil
1 large mango, diced
2 kiwifruit, peeled and diced
½ cup peeled, seeded, and diced cucumber
⅓ cup quartered grape tomatoes
⅓ cup minced red onion
⅓ cup chopped celery

Dressing
3 tablespoons freshly squeezed lime juice
1 tablespoon honey
1 teaspoon salt-free Caribbean Citrus seasoning
½ teaspoon fresh lime zest
4 tablespoons olive oil

4 cups mixed greens

Garnish
Toasted slivered almonds (optional)

1. Prepare the shrimp: In a large bowl, combine the Caribbean Citrus seasoning with the shrimp and toss to coat.

2. Heat the canola oil in a large skillet over medium-high heat. Add the shrimp in two batches and sauté on both sides for about 3 minutes per side, or until cooked through.

3. Meanwhile, combine the mango, kiwifruit, cucumber, grape tomatoes, red onion, and celery in a large bowl. Add the cooked shrimp to the bowl.

4. Prepare the dressing: In a small bowl, whisk together the lime juice, honey, Caribbean Citrus seasoning, and lime zest. In a thin stream, add the olive oil, whisking constantly to emulsify. Pour the dressing over the salad.

5. Line a platter with the mixed greens. Pile the shrimp salad on top of the greens. Garnish with toasted slivered almonds if desired.

Sichuan Lamb

6 SERVINGS/SERVING SIZE: 2 LAMB LOINS

PREPARATION TIME: 10 MINUTES

COOK TIME: 20 MINUTES

When I first learned how to prepare lamb, it was a basic method, with perhaps just some garlic, salt, and pepper. But lamb's gaminess can really take on more assertive flavors. I found that out when developing this bold recipe using a quartet of Asian-inspired ingredients. Chinese five-spice powder, coriander, Sichuan peppercorns, and white pepper take lamb to new heights. No salt needed!

3 tablespoons toasted sesame oil
2 tablespoons canola oil
1 teaspoon Chinese five-spice powder
1 teaspoon ground coriander
1 teaspoon ground Sichuan peppercorns or ground smoked black pepper
1 teaspoon white pepper
2 garlic cloves, minced finely
12 lamb loin chops, about 2 inches thick, trimmed of excess fat

1. In a shallow baking dish, combine the sesame oil, canola oil, Chinese five-spice powder, coriander, Sichuan pepper, white pepper, and garlic.

CORIANDER

Coriander seeds are the seeds of the cilantro plant, and are one of the oldest known spices. Romans used coriander to preserve meat and to flavor wine. The taste and smell of coriander seeds and cilantro leaves are different but complement each other. The seeds and leaves are often used together to provide complexity of flavor in a meat dish.

2. Place the lamb loins in a shallow baking pan. Pour the spice mixture over the lamb and rub on both sides of each lamb loin. Cover and refrigerate for 2 hours. Remove the lamb from the refrigerator and let come to room temperature for 20 minutes.

3. Prepare an outdoor grill. Coat the grill rack with cooking spray. Heat the grill to medium-high and grill the lamb for 4 to 7 minutes per side for medium rare (about 145°F on an instant-read thermometer).

4. Remove the lamb from the grill and let rest for a few minutes before serving.

Lamb Korma

4 SERVINGS/SERVING SIZE: ½ CUP

PREPARATION TIME: 10 MINUTES

COOK TIME: 65 TO 95 MINUTES

Sometimes it really is okay to indulge a little. I wanted to include a few recipes that you might not eat every day, but would save for a special occasion. Lamb Korma is one of those traditional Indian recipes where it is worth sticking with a tried-and-true formula of rich ingredients. Ginger and garam masala carry the dish, so no salt is needed.

● ● ● ● ● ● ● ● ●

1¼ cups whole-milk yogurt
2 large onions, chopped
1 (2-inch) piece of fresh ginger, peeled and chopped
2 tablespoons garam masala
½ cup heavy cream
1 pound lean boneless lamb loin, cut into 1-inch cubes
½ cup toasted unsalted cashew pieces
¼ cup golden raisins

Garnish
2 tablespoons minced fresh cilantro

1. Place the yogurt, onions, and ginger in a food processor or blender. Puree until smooth.

2. In a large Dutch oven, combine the puree, garam masala, cream, and lamb. Bring to a very gentle boil, cover the pot, and simmer over low heat for 1 to 1½ hours. Check occasionally to be sure the mixture is not sticking to the bottom of the pan.

3. Add the cashews and raisins and cook for another 5 minutes. Serve over rice if desired. Garnish with the cilantro.

DID YOU KNOW?
Reduced-fat versions of ingredients usually make up for the flavor loss by adding sugar or salt. Slashing 40 calories may not be worth all that extra sodium!

BASIC NUTRITIONAL VALUES
Calories 455
　Calories from Fat 245
Total Fat 27.0 g
　Saturated Fat 12.0 g
　Trans Fat 0 g
Cholesterol 110 mg
Sodium 120 mg
Total Carbohydrate 30 g
　Dietary Fiber 4 g
　Sugars 15 g
Protein 27 g

Classic Steak au Poivre

2 SERVINGS/SERVING SIZE: 1 STEAK

PREPARATION TIME: 5 MINUTES

COOK TIME: 8 MINUTES

I love recipes where one spice or herb carries the entire dish. Peppercorns can lay claim to that honor, as they are the star of this classic. No surprises here, just perfect flavor with the crunch and heat of fabulous pepper.

❀ ❀ ❀ ❀ ❀ ❀ ❀ ❀ ❀

2 filets mignons (4 to 5 ounces each)
1 tablespoon black peppercorns
1 tablespoon unsalted butter
2 tablespoons canola oil
2 tablespoons cognac
⅓ cup crème fraîche

1. Pat the steaks dry and let them rest at room temperature for 30 minutes prior to cooking. Coarsely crush the peppercorns, using either a mortar and pestle or a spice grinder.

2. Coat each side of each steak with the peppercorns.

3. Melt the butter and oil in a large, heavy-bottomed skillet. When the butter is sizzling, add the steaks and cook for about 4 minutes per side, until crusty.

4. Remove the skillet from the heat. Pour off any excess fat from the skillet. Heat the cognac in a small skillet and let it reduce for about 1 minute. When warm, pour the cognac over the steaks. Transfer the steaks to a warm plate.

5. Add the crème fraîche to the skillet and bring to a boil, scraping up the browned bits. Whisk the sauce and pour over the steaks.

BASIC NUTRITIONAL VALUES

Calories 425
  Calories from Fat 295
Total Fat 33.0 g
  Saturated Fat 14.0 g
  Trans Fat 0 g
Cholesterol 120 mg
Sodium 60 mg
Total Carbohydrate 3 g
  Dietary Fiber 1 g
  Sugars 0 g
Protein 22 g

Herb Frittata

6 SERVINGS/SERVING SIZE: ⅙ PAN

PREPARATION TIME: 10 MINUTES

COOK TIME: 25 MINUTES

One dish that is the perfect place to showcase herbs is the frittata. Here I've combined fresh chives and basil with a kick from Lemon Pepper seasoning that makes these eggs anything but your usual Sunday morning breakfast. Try all sorts of herbs, such as dill, thyme, sage, or tarragon—they all work beautifully.

● ● ● ● ● ● ● ● ●

1 tablespoon plus 1 teaspoon olive oil
1 tablespoon unsalted butter
6 ounces sliced cremini mushrooms, stemmed
¼ teaspoon red pepper flakes
½ cup diced onion
2 garlic cloves, minced
½ cup rehydrated sliced sun-dried tomatoes (not oil-packed)
6 eggs, beaten
2 tablespoons fat-free milk
2 tablespoons chopped fresh chives
1 tablespoon chopped fresh basil
½ teaspoon salt-free Lemon Pepper seasoning
2 tablespoons freshly grated Parmesan cheese

1. Heat the 1 tablespoon of the olive oil and butter in a large, ovenproof skillet over medium-high heat. Add the mushrooms, in two batches if necessary so that the mushrooms sauté in one layer, and red pepper flakes and sauté until the mushrooms are browned. Remove the mushrooms from the skillet and set aside.

2. Add the remaining 1 teaspoon of olive oil to the skillet and add the onion and garlic. Sauté for 4 to 5 minutes over medium heat. Add the sun-dried tomatoes and sauté for 2 minutes.

3. Preheat the oven to broil. Set the rack 6 inches from the heat source. Beat the eggs with the milk in a large bowl. Add the chives, basil, and Lemon Pepper seasoning. Add the mushrooms back to the skillet with the onion and pour the eggs over the vegetables. Let the eggs cook undisturbed for 2 to 3 minutes. Lift the edges of the frittata with a spatula to let the uncooked portion of the eggs flow to the bottom. Continue to cook until eggs are almost set.

4. Sprinkle the top of the frittata with Parmesan cheese. Transfer the skillet to the oven, set under the broiler. Broil the frittata until the cheese melts and the eggs are just set. Cut into wedges to serve.

BASIC NUTRITIONAL VALUES

Calories 150
Calories from Fat 90
Total Fat 10.0 g
Saturated Fat 3.5 g
Trans Fat 0 g
Cholesterol 195 mg
Sodium 175 mg
Total Carbohydrate 6 g
Dietary Fiber 1 g
Sugars 3 g
Protein 9 g

Mango Cashew Chicken Bundles with Sesame Quinoa

MAKES 8 SERVINGS, 1 BUNDLE PER
  SERVING

PREPARATION TIME: 1 HOUR
  (INCLUDING MARINATING TIME)

COOK TIME: 15 MINUTES

A take-off on traditional Asian lettuce wraps, these bundles benefit from fiber and protein-rich quinoa and crunchy cashews.

❧ ❧ ❧ ❧ ❧ ❧ ❧ ❧

BASIC NUTRITIONAL VALUES

Calories 370
  Calories from Fat 190
Total Fat 21.0 g
  Saturated Fat 4.0 g
  Trans Fat 0 g
Cholesterol 35 mg
Sodium 115 mg
Total Carbohydrate 30 g
  Dietary Fiber 4 g
  Sugars 9 g
Protein 17 g

6   boneless, skinless chicken thighs, cut into 1-inch cubes
2   tablespoons canola oil
1½ tablespoons minced fresh ginger
1   tablespoon reduced-sodium soy sauce
1   tablespoon honey
1   cup uncooked quinoa, well rinsed and drained
1   tablespoon sesame oil
¼   cup sesame seeds, toasted
⅓   cup diced onion
4   garlic cloves
1   cup diced mango (about 1 mango)
1   cup unsalted cashews
½   cup chopped fresh cilantro
8   iceberg lettuce leaves

1. Combine the chicken, 1 tablespoon of the oil, and the ginger, soy sauce, and honey in a bowl. Marinate in the refrigerator at least 30 minutes.

2. Cook the quinoa according to the package directions. Stir in the sesame oil and toasted sesame seeds. Cover and set aside.

3. Place the remaining tablespoon of canola oil in a skillet and heat over medium-high heat. Add the onion and cook until translucent, about 5 minutes. Add the garlic and cook until aromatic, about 1 minute. Add the chicken with its marinade and brown it on all sides, 8 to 10 minutes. Stir in the mango and cashews and heat until warm. Remove from the heat and stir in the cilantro.

4. Let the chicken mixture cool briefly. To create the bundles, wrap a tablespoonful of quinoa and a tablespoonful of the chicken mixture in a lettuce leaf to make a small pouch being careful to not overstuff. Serve warm.

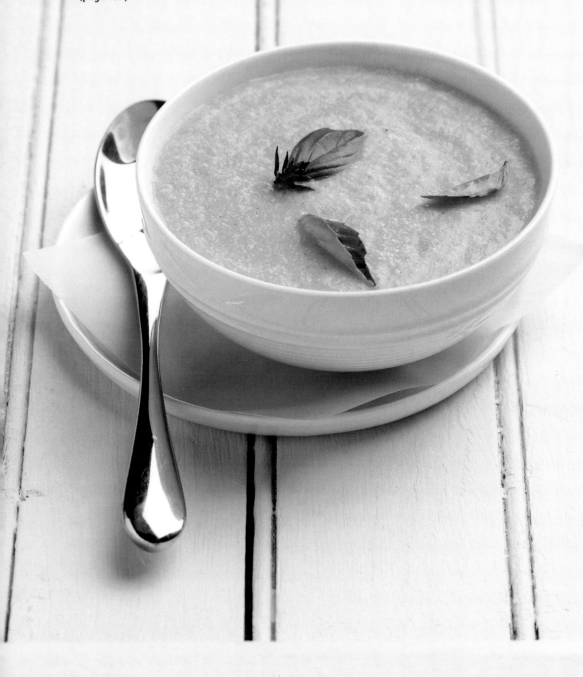

CHINESE FIVE-SPICE MELON SOUP

(page 137)

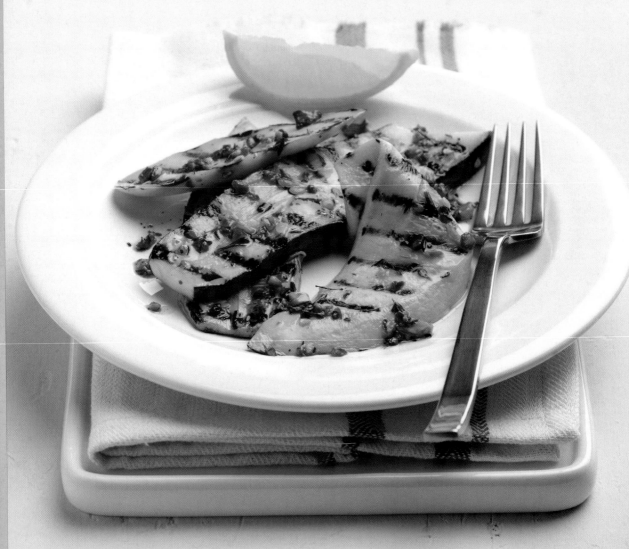

HERBES DE PROVENCE SQUASH

(page 109)

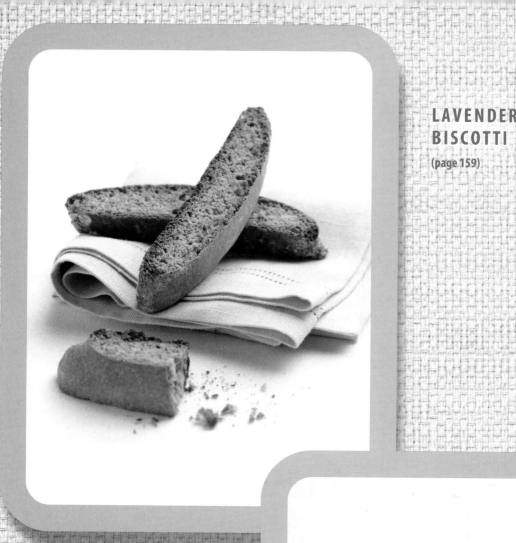

LAVENDER
BISCOTTI
(page 159)

LEMON THYME
FRUIT SALAD
(page 157)

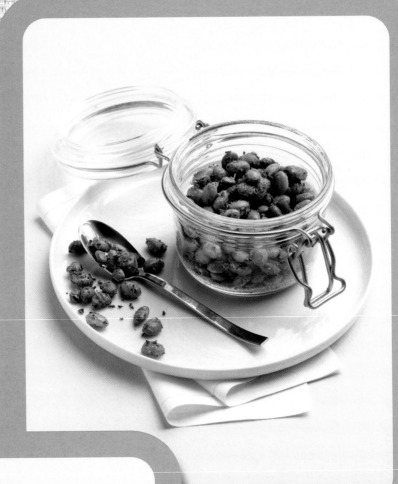

**ROASTED
ITALIAN
EDAMAME**

(page 25)

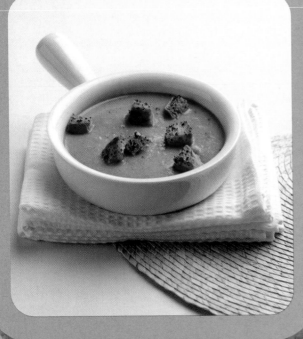

**ITALIAN ROASTED
RED PEPPER SOUP
WITH GARLIC CROUTONS**

(page 124)

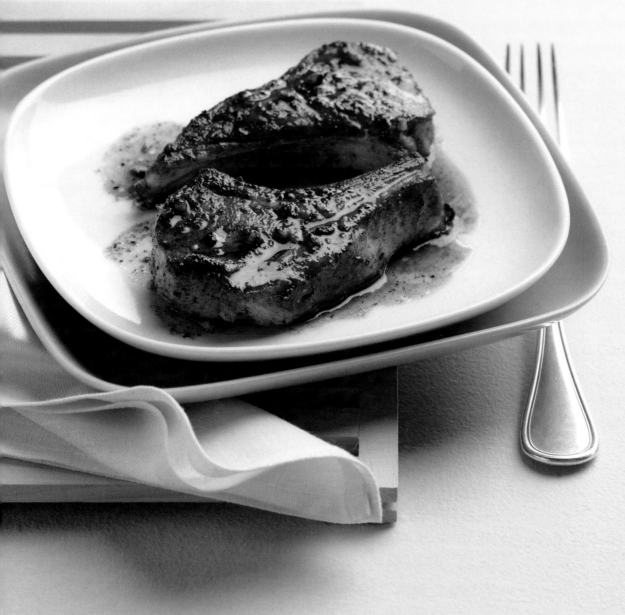

SICHUAN LAMB (page 79)

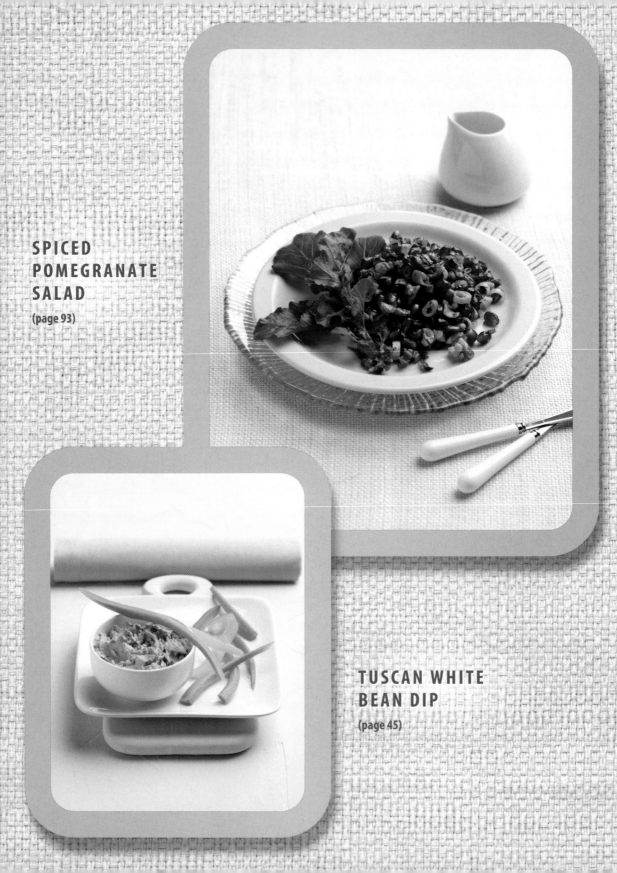

**SPICED
POMEGRANATE
SALAD**

(page 93)

**TUSCAN WHITE
BEAN DIP**

(page 45)

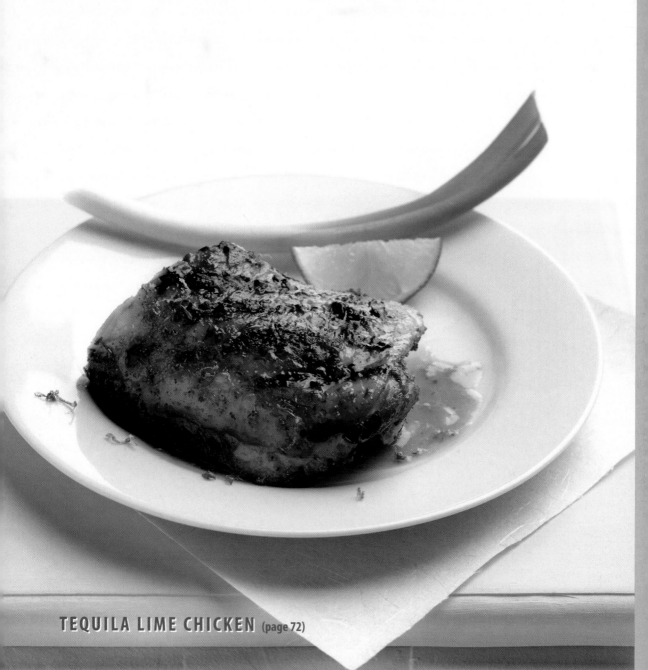

TEQUILA LIME CHICKEN (page 72)

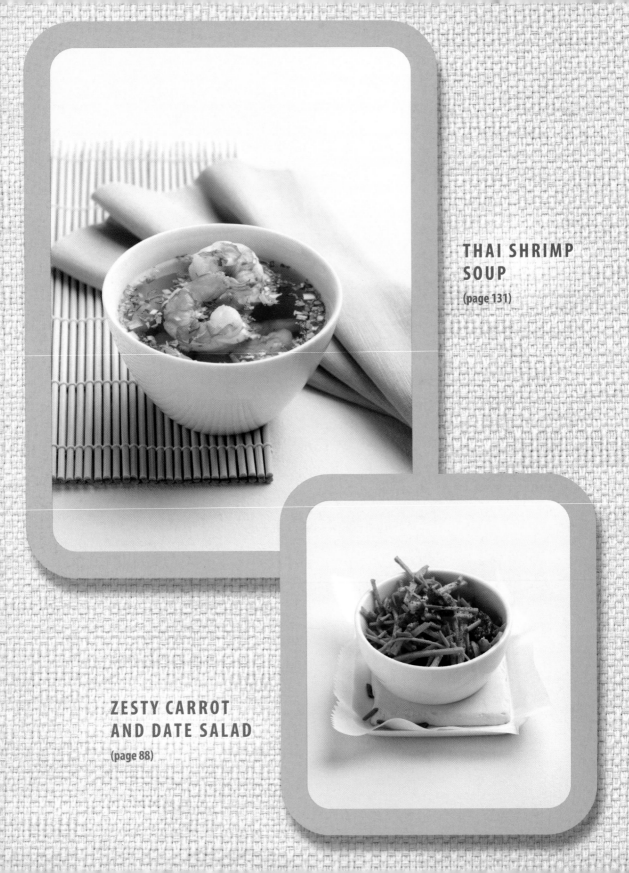

THAI SHRIMP SOUP

(page 131)

ZESTY CARROT AND DATE SALAD

(page 88)

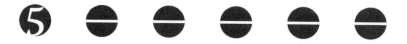

Sides

New Potatoes with Creamy Italian Herb Dressing

6 SERVINGS/SERVING SIZE: ½ CUP

PREPARATION TIME: 12 MINUTES

COOK TIME: 25 MINUTES

Boiled potatoes always make a great side dish, but frankly they can be a little boring all by themselves. So I've come up with luscious, silky dressing to coat the potatoes in scented herbs. This recipe is so good with either dried Italian seasoning or fresh herbs, I couldn't resist giving you both versions.

❀ ❀ ❀ ❀ ❀ ❀ ❀ ❀

½ cup light mayonnaise (such as Hellmann's)
2 teaspoons salt-free Italian seasoning
½ cup 1% fat buttermilk
2 tablespoons cider vinegar
¼ teaspoon freshly ground black pepper
½ teaspoon hot sauce, or to taste
2 pounds small new potatoes, unpeeled, scrubbed well

1. Combine the mayonnaise and Italian seasoning in a small bowl. Whisk well. Slowly whisk in the buttermilk, cider vinegar, black pepper, and hot sauce. Cover and refrigerate for 30 minutes.

2. Meanwhile, steam the potatoes. Pour about 1 inch of water into a large pot or Dutch oven. Place a steamer basket inside the pot. Place the potatoes in the steamer and steam for 20 to 25 minutes, adding water as necessary to prevent the pot from drying out. Steam until a tester is easily inserted into a potato. Cut each potato in half and serve with the Creamy Italian Herb dressing.

DID YOU KNOW?

Surface salt is more noticeable than salt that is already in processed foods. Although a handful of salted peanuts might seem really salty, they contain slightly less sodium than does a cup of dairy milk.

To Use Fresh Herbs for This Recipe
Combine 1/4 cup of loosely packed fresh parsley leaves, 2 tablespoons of coarsely chopped fresh oregano leaves, 2 tablespoons of coarsely chopped fresh basil, and 1 teaspoon of minced fresh rosemary with the mayonnaise in a food processor. Process until the herbs are chopped. Slowly add the buttermilk, vinegar, black pepper, and hot sauce until combined.

BASIC NUTRITIONAL VALUES

Calories 210
  Calories from Fat 45
Total Fat 5.0 g
  Saturated Fat 1.0 g
  Trans Fat 0 g
Cholesterol 5 mg
Sodium 200 mg
Total Carbohydrate 37 g
  Dietary Fiber 3 g
  Sugars 4 g
Protein 4 g

Linguine with Walnuts and Garlic and Herbs

6 SERVINGS/SERVING SIZE: 1¼ CUPS

PREPARATION TIME: 10 MINUTES

COOK TIME: 30 MINUTES

With essentially only four ingredients, this is the perfect side dish or main dish. The Garlic & Herb seasoning and walnuts make a powerful flavor duo, while the olive oil coats each strand of pasta with a silky texture. Be sure to use good-quality olive oil.

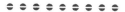

1 pound linguine
⅓ cup olive oil
½ cup coarsely chopped walnuts
2 teaspoons salt-free Garlic & Herb seasoning
  Freshly ground black pepper

1. Cook the pasta according to the package directions, omitting the salt, until al dente. Drain, reserving about ¼ cup of the pasta water.

2. Meanwhile, heat the oil in a large skillet over medium heat. Add the walnuts and toast for 1 to 2 minutes. Add the Garlic & Herb seasoning. Cook for about 1 minute. Add the reserved pasta water. Cook for 2 minutes. Add the drained pasta and coat well. Finish with freshly ground black pepper.

To Cook This Recipe with Fresh Garlic and Herbs
Heat the oil and garlic together over medium-low heat for about 4 minutes, until the garlic is fragrant but not browned. Add the walnuts and toast for 3 minutes. Add the reserved pasta water, 2 tablespoons of minced fresh basil, and 2 tablespoons of minced fresh parsley. Add the drained pasta and toss well. Season with freshly ground black pepper.

BASIC NUTRITIONAL VALUES

Calories 465
Calories from Fat 180
Total Fat 20.0 g
Saturated Fat 2.5 g
Trans Fat 0 g
Cholesterol 0 mg
Sodium 0 mg
Total Carbohydrate 59 g
Dietary Fiber 4 g
Sugars 1 g
Protein 12 g

Zesty Carrot and Date Salad

4 SERVINGS/SERVING SIZE: 1 CUP

PREPARATION TIME: 20 MINUTES

COOK TIME: 0

As an alternative to a predictable shredded or chopped carrot salad, I chose to make elegant julienne strips of bright orange, crunchy carrots. The tandoori-style seasoning further enhances the bright color of this salad, and juicy, sweet dates give this anytime salad an exotic twist.

⊜ ⊜ ⊜ ⊜ ⊜ ⊜ ⊜ ⊜

6 large carrots (1 pound), peeled and cut into thin julienne (5 cups)
1¼ teaspoons salt-free tandoori-style seasoning
1 large garlic clove, minced to a paste
3 tablespoons freshly squeezed lemon juice
⅓ cup olive oil
½ cup sliced pitted dates
Freshly ground black pepper
2 tablespoons minced fresh chives

1. Place the carrots in a salad bowl and set aside.

2. In a small bowl, whisk together the tandoori-style seasoning with the garlic and lemon juice. Slowly add the olive oil in a thin stream, whisking constantly, until the dressing is emulsified.

3. Add the dressing to the carrots and add the dates. Mix well.

4. Let the salad stand at room temperature for 30 minutes prior to serving. Plate each salad and garnish with freshly ground black pepper and chopped chives.

BASIC NUTRITIONAL VALUES

Calories 255
  Calories from Fat 160
Total Fat 18.0 g
  Saturated Fat 2.5 g
  Trans Fat 0 g
Cholesterol 0 mg
Sodium 75 mg
Total Carbohydrate 25 g
  Dietary Fiber 5 g
  Sugars 17 g
Protein 2 g

Lemon Pepper Barley Pilaf

5 SERVINGS/SERVING SIZE: ½ CUP

PREPARATION TIME: 15 MINUTES

COOK TIME: 60 MINUTES

Barley needs more respect. Often relegated to just being used in soup, barley receives its due with this salad. The subtle lemon flavor permeating throughout this any-season salad neither overwhelms nor detracts from its nutty flavor.

❂ ❂ ❂ ❂ ❂ ❂ ❂ ❂ ❂

BASIC NUTRITIONAL VALUES

Calories 300
  Calories from Fat 80
Total Fat 9.0 g
  Saturated Fat 1.5 g
  Trans Fat 0 g
Cholesterol 0 mg
Sodium 55 mg
Total Carbohydrate 48 g
  Dietary Fiber 8 g
  Sugars 9 g
Protein 9 g

1 tablespoon olive oil
1 large onion, chopped
1 cup pearl barley
1 teaspoon salt-free Lemon Pepper seasoning*
2½ cups low-sodium, reduced-fat chicken stock (page 123)
½ cup coarsely chopped raw cashews
1 tablespoon freshly squeezed lemon juice
⅓ cup golden raisins
2 tablespoons minced fresh parsley

Garnish
¼ cup seeded and finely minced red bell pepper

1. Heat the oil in a heavy skillet over medium heat. Add the onion and sauté for 7 to 8 minutes, until lightly browned. Add the barley and toast for 1 minute. Add the Lemon Pepper seasoning and sauté for 1 minute. Pour in the stock and bring to a boil.

2. Lower the heat to low, cover, and simmer the barley for about 40 minutes, until almost all the liquid is absorbed.

3. Toast the cashew pieces in a dry skillet until lightly browned.

4. Add the lemon juice and raisins to the barley. Remove the saucepan from the heat and let the mixture stand for 5 minutes. Add the cashews and parsley and toss gently. Garnish with minced red bell pepper.

Instead of Using the Lemon Pepper Seasoning
Substitute 1 teaspoon of grated fresh lemon zest and ¼ teaspoon of freshly ground black pepper.

Goat Cheese Penne with Garlic and Herbs

6 SERVINGS/SERVING SIZE: 1⅓ CUPS

PREPARATION TIME: 5 MINUTES

COOK TIME: 20 MINUTES

Garlic and cherry tomatoes are always a winning combination that I use often in my cooking. This is really two recipes in one. Try serving just the garlic-scented cherry tomatoes as a side to any dish, or continue further with the recipe in its entirety. The nooks and crannies of the penne capture the creamy herb sauce. Any similarly shaped pasta will do the same.

❧ ❧ ❧ ❧ ❧ ❧ ❧ ❧ ❧

2   cups halved cherry tomatoes
1   tablespoon salt-free Garlic & Herb seasoning*
1   tablespoon olive oil
1   pound whole wheat or white penne noodles
½   cup mild goat cheese
¼   cup part-skim ricotta cheese
¼   cup sliced fresh basil
¼   cup minced fresh oregano

1. Preheat the oven to 400°F. Line a baking sheet with parchment paper and set aside. In a medium-size bowl, toss the cherry tomatoes with the Garlic & Herb seasoning and olive oil. Mix until well coated.

2. Spread the tomatoes in a single layer on the prepared baking sheet. Roast the tomatoes for about 20 minutes, until lightly browned.

3. Meanwhile, bring a large pot of water to a boil. Add the penne and cook until al dente, 7 to 9 minutes. Drain, reserving about ⅓ cup of the pasta water.

4. Place the goat cheese and ricotta cheese in a medium-size bowl. Add the reserved cooking water from the pasta and whisk well. Add the roasted cherry tomatoes and drained pasta, and toss well. Garnish with fresh basil and oregano.

> **DID YOU KNOW?**
> An ounce of whole milk ricotta cheese contains 24 milligrams of sodium, an ounce of grated Parmesan contains 152 milligrams, and an ounce of processed cheese contains as much as 410 milligrams!

To make this recipe with fresh herbs and garlic
Toss the cherry tomatoes with 2 finely minced fresh garlic cloves and 2 tablespoons of either fresh oregano or basil or a combination of the two. Proceed to roast the cherry tomatoes as directed. Garnish with additional fresh herbs if desired.

BASIC NUTRITIONAL VALUES

Calories 385
  Calories from Fat 80
Total Fat 9.0 g
  Saturated Fat 4.0 g
  Trans Fat 0 g
Cholesterol 15 mg
Sodium 70 mg
Total Carbohydrate 63 g
  Dietary Fiber 9 g
  Sugars 5 g
Protein 15 g

Penne with Salsa Cruda

12 SERVINGS/SERVING SIZE: 1 CUP

COOK TIME: 20 MINUTES

PREPARATION TIME: 10 MINUTES

This is like having bruschetta over pasta instead of bread! The cool flavors are light and fresh, perfect for a summer side dish. When heirloom tomatoes are at their height, try using them in this dish. An abundance of differently colored tomatoes look beautiful against the pasta and green herbs.

❀ ❀ ❀ ❀ ❀ ❀ ❀ ❀ ❀

1 pound penne
1½ pounds large ripe tomatoes
2 garlic cloves, minced
3 tablespoons olive oil
1 tablespoon salt-free Italian seasoning
¼ cup sliced fresh basil
2 tablespoons thinly sliced scallions

Garnish
Freshly ground black pepper
Hot sauce or crushed red pepper flakes

1. Bring a large pot of water to a rapid boil. Add the penne and cook until al dente, 7 to 8 minutes. Drain the pasta well.

2. While the pasta is cooking, cut the tomatoes across and remove the seeds. Dice the tomatoes and place in a large serving bowl. Combine the tomatoes with the garlic, 2 tablespoons of the olive oil, and the Italian seasoning, fresh basil, and scallions. Mix well.

3. Toss the remaining tablespoon of olive oil with the cooked penne. Mix in black pepper and crushed red pepper or hot sauce just to taste. Mix the salsa cruda with the cooked penne and serve.

BASIC NUTRITIONAL VALUES

Calories 175
  Calories from Fat 35
Total Fat 4.0 g
  Saturated Fat 0.5 g
  Trans Fat 0 g
Cholesterol 0 mg
Sodium 0 mg
Total Carbohydrate 30 g
  Dietary Fiber 2 g
  Sugars 2 g
Protein 5 g

Fresh Peas and Zucchini

8 SERVINGS/SERVING SIZE: ½ CUP

PREPARATION TIME: 20 MINUTES

COOK TIME: 25 MINUTES

Fresh peas are such a treat that I cringe when I find peas drowned in cream, butter, or cheese. Here I combine them with farm-fresh tomatoes and zucchini and let the all-purpose seasoning carry all the sweet flavor of fresh peas.

❂ ❂ ❂ ❂ ❂ ❂ ❂ ❂ ❂

3 tablespoons olive oil
6 scallions, chopped
2 cups fresh peas
3 large tomatoes, seeded and diced
2 teaspoons no-salt all-purpose seasoning
⅔ cup water
4 small zucchini, sliced diagonally into ½-inch slices

1. Heat 2 tablespoons of the oil in a large skillet. Add the scallions and sauté for 1 to 2 minutes, until glistening. Add the peas and tomatoes and cook for 3 minutes.

2. Add the all-purpose seasoning and sauté for 1 minute. Add the water and zucchini and cook for about 20 minutes over low heat. Drizzle the remaining tablespoon of olive oil on top of the vegetables and serve.

BASIC NUTRITIONAL VALUES

Calories 105
  Calories from Fat 45
Total Fat 5.0 g
  Saturated Fat 1.0 g
  Trans Fat 0 g
Cholesterol 0 mg
Sodium 10 mg
Total Carbohydrate 12 g
  Dietary Fiber 4 g
  Sugars 5 g
Protein 4 g

Spiced Pomegranate Salad

4 SERVINGS/SERVING SIZE: ½ CUP (NOT INCLUDING GREENS)

PREPARATION TIME: 15 MINUTES

COOK TIME: 5 MINUTES

Salad doesn't have to equal lettuce and a few random slices of tomato and cucumber. This spiced pomegranate salad combines juicy and sweet pomegranate seeds with toasted walnuts, fresh scallions, and parsley. A bit of delightful heat comes from the Southwest Chipotle seasoning. Between the sweet and heat, there is no need for salt!

❀ ❀ ❀ ❀ ❀ ❀ ❀ ❀

½ cup coarsely chopped walnuts
3 scallions, chopped
   Seeds and juice of 1 large pomegranate
3 tablespoons olive oil
1 teaspoon salt-free Southwest Chipotle seasoning
3 tablespoons minced fresh parsley
4 cups mixed greens

1. Toast the walnuts in a large skillet over medium heat until lightly browned, shaking the pan occasionally. Watch carefully so the nuts do not burn. Transfer the toasted walnuts to a bowl.

2. Add the remaining ingredients to the nuts and toss. Serve over mixed greens.

PARSLEY
There are two main varieties of parsley, flat-leaf (a.k.a. Italian) and curly. Flat-leaf parsley is often preferred for use in recipes, whereas curly parsley is often used as a garnish. Parsley is a very good source of vitamins A and C.

BASIC NUTRITIONAL VALUE

Calories 265
  Calories from Fat 190
Total Fat 21.0 g
  Saturated Fat 2.5 g
  Trans Fat 0 g
Cholesterol 0 mg
Sodium 20 mg
Total Carbohydrate 19 g
  Dietary Fiber 5 g
  Sugars 12 g
Protein 4 g

Cherry Tomato and Avocado Salad

14 SERVINGS/SERVING SIZE: ½ CUP

PREPARATION TIME: 20 MINUTES

COOK TIME: 0

I used to make tomato and avocado sandwiches all the time. Now that I've cut down my bread consumption, I've deconstructed the sandwich into a salad. Silky avocado combines with crunchy cucumber, pungent yet sweet red onion, and ripe cherry tomatoes for an easy warm-weather salad.

☙ ☙ ☙ ☙ ☙ ☙ ☙ ☙ ☙

Salad
2 pints cherry or grape tomatoes, halved
1 large avocado, peeled, pitted, and cut into ½-inch cubes
1 small cucumber, peeled, seeded, and diced into ½-inch pieces
½ small red onion, sliced thinly

Vinaigrette
3 tablespoons olive oil
2 tablespoons freshly squeezed lemon juice
1½ tablespoons balsamic vinegar
2 teaspoons salt-free Italian seasoning
1 teaspoon minced garlic
Pinch of sugar

Garnish
¼ cup sliced fresh basil

1. Combine the tomatoes, avocado, cucumber, and red onion in a serving bowl.

2. Whisk together the vinaigrette ingredients and add to the cherry tomato mixture. Toss well and let stand at room temperature for 30 minutes prior to serving.

3. Garnish the salad with fresh basil.

BASIC NUTRITIONAL VALUES

Calories 60
  Calories from Fat 45
Total Fat 5.0 g
  Saturated Fat 0.5 g
  Trans Fat 0 g
Cholesterol 0 mg
Sodium 0 mg
Total Carbohydrate 4 g
  Dietary Fiber 2 g
  Sugars 2 g
Protein 1 g

Sugar Snap Peas with Pecans

8 SERVINGS/SERVING SIZE: ½ CUP

PREPARATION TIME: 12 MINUTES

COOK TIME: 10 MINUTES

Usually sugar snap peas show up in stir-fries. I like to prepare them simply, sautéed quickly with some Garlic & Herb seasoning, a touch of shallots, and a crunchy nut topping. Let the sugar snaps take center stage and fuss with them as little as possible.

✻ ✻ ✻ ✻ ✻ ✻ ✻ ✻

¼ cup chopped pecans
2 teaspoons olive oil
1 small shallot, minced
1 teaspoon salt-free Garlic & Herb seasoning
1 pound fresh sugar snap peas, trimmed
2 tablespoons water

Garnish
2 teaspoons grated fresh lemon zest

1. Place the pecans in a dry 10-inch skillet and toast them over medium heat, stirring occasionally, about 4 minutes. Remove the pecans from the skillet and set aside. Heat the olive oil in the same skillet over medium heat. Add the shallot and sauté for 2 minutes. Add the Garlic & Herb Seasoning and sauté for 1 minute.

2. Add the sugar snap peas and sauté for 1 minute. Add the water, then cover and steam for 4 minutes, or until the sugar snap peas turn bright green and are crisp.

3. Garnish the sugar snap peas with the pecans. Sprinkle with fresh lemon zest.

BASIC NUTRITIONAL VALUES

Calories 65
  Calories from Fat 35
Total Fat 4.0 g
  Saturated Fat 0 g
  Trans Fat 0 g
Cholesterol 0 mg
Sodium 5 mg
Total Carbohydrate 6 g
  Dietary Fiber 2 g
  Sugars 2 g
Protein 2 g

Italian Greens

4 SERVINGS/SERVING SIZE: ⅔ CUP

PREPARATION TIME: 10 MINUTES

COOK TIME: 8 TO 10 MINUTES

We all know we should eat more greens. But who can face boring salads of lettuce night after night? Fortunately the healthiest greens are ones you typically have to cook. With the enhancement of Italian seasoning and a drizzle of really good balsamic vinegar, you'll be eating greens often. This side dish goes well with a simple grilled lean steak.

≋ ≋ ≋ ≋ ≋ ≋ ≋ ≋

1	large head escarole, washed gently and patted dry
10	ounces fresh baby spinach leaves, stems removed, washed gently and patted dry
3	tablespoons pine nuts
2	tablespoons olive oil
4	garlic cloves, slivered
2	teaspoons salt-free Italian seasoning
¼	teaspoon sugar
⅛	teaspoon crushed red chili flakes
1	tablespoon good-quality balsamic vinegar

1. Core the escarole, discard any bruised or browned leaves, and wash thoroughly. Drain and pat dry. Tear the escarole into large pieces. Discard any spinach leaves that are yellow or wilted.

2. Toast the pine nuts in a 12-inch dry skillet over medium heat until lightly browned, shaking the pan occasionally. Watch carefully so the nuts do not burn. Transfer the toasted pine nuts to a bowl.

3. Heat the olive oil in the same 12-inch skillet over medium heat. Add the garlic and sauté for 1 to 2 minutes, until lightly golden. Add the Italian seasoning, sugar, and crushed red pepper and shake the pan to disperse the seasonings. Add the escarole and spinach and turn the leaves with a set of tongs until they begin to wilt. Cover the pan and cook for 2 to 3 minutes.

4. Sprinkle the vinegar over the greens and stir. Garnish with toasted pine nuts.

BASIC NUTRITIONAL VALUES

Calories 145
  Calories from Fat 110
Total Fat 12.0 g
  Saturated Fat 1.5 g
  Trans Fat 0 g
Cholesterol 0 mg
Sodium 80 mg
Total Carbohydrate 9 g
  Dietary Fiber 5 g
  Sugars 2 g
Protein 4 g

Okra with Onions

4 SERVINGS/SERVING SIZE: 1 CUP

PREPARATION TIME: 10 MINUTES

COOK TIME: 22 MINUTES

The first time I ate okra was not in the southern United States, even though it is most popular there. No, it was in an Indian restaurant, and I was hooked right then and there. This is okra beefed up with tandoori-style spice and sautéed until tender but with a crunch that remains. If you think you don't like okra, you are probably reacting to the unpleasant texture that results from its being stewed for so long, as it often is. Here, the texture is right on the mark.

1 pound fresh okra, washed and ends trimmed
1 teaspoon whole cumin seeds
2 tablespoons canola oil
1½ teaspoons salt-free tandoori-style seasoning
1 medium-size onion, halved and sliced thinly
  Freshly ground black pepper

1. Cut each okra in half on the diagonal.

2. Place the cumin seeds in a large skillet and toast for 1 to 2 minutes. Add 1 tablespoon of the oil and the tandoori-style seasoning and cook for 30 seconds. Add the onion and sauté over medium heat for 6 to 8 minutes.

3. Add the remaining 5 teaspoons of oil to the skillet. Add the okra and cook for 5 to 7 minutes. Add the freshly ground black pepper and continue to cook for 5 to 6 minutes more, until the okra is cooked through but still slightly crunchy.

BASIC NUTRITIONAL VALUES

Calories 120
  Calories from Fat 65
Total Fat 7.0 g
  Saturated Fat 0.5 g
  Trans Fat 0 g
Cholesterol 0 mg
Sodium 10 mg
Total Carbohydrate 12 g
  Dietary Fiber 3 g
  Sugars 4 g
Protein 3 g

Herbed Mashed Potatoes with Olive Oil

8 SERVINGS/SERVING SIZE: ½ CUP

PREPARATION TIME: 15 MINUTES

COOK TIME: 40 MINUTES

Forget the blue cheese, bacon, and anything else you do to jazz up potatoes. These potatoes are just the purest form of a good mash. Rich olive oil, sprinkles of Italian seasoning, and some of the starchy water to mash the potatoes are all that's needed for a satisfying side.

⊜ ⊜ ⊜ ⊜ ⊜ ⊜ ⊜ ⊜

2 pounds baking potatoes, peeled and cut into quarters
⅓ cup olive oil
2 teaspoons salt-free Italian seasoning
   Freshly ground black or white pepper

1. Bring a large pot of water to a boil. Add the potatoes and simmer, partially covered, for about 20 minutes, or until the potatoes are soft.

2. Drain the potatoes, reserving about ½ cup of the warm cooking water in a bowl. Place the potatoes back in the pot and cover the pot with a towel and then a lid. Let the potatoes stand for 10 minutes.

3. Meanwhile, add the olive oil, Italian seasoning, and freshly ground black or white pepper to the reserved cooking water. Add the olive oil mixture to the potatoes and, using a potato masher, mash to a soft puree. Taste and adjust the seasoning.

> **DID YOU KNOW?**
> Instead of a salt shaker, keep a shaker of no-salt all-purpose seasoning on the dinner table.

BASIC NUTRITIONAL VALUES

Calories 155
  Calories from Fat 80
Total Fat 9.0 g
  Saturated Fat 1.5 g
  Trans Fat 0 g
Cholesterol 0 mg
Sodium 0 mg
Total Carbohydrate 18 g
  Dietary Fiber 2 g
  Sugars 1 g
Protein 2 g

Wild Rice with Herbs and Mushrooms

8 SERVINGS/SERVING SIZE: ½ CUP

TIME: 15 MINUTES

COOK TIME: 25 MINUTES

Want to look like you slaved all day in the kitchen? This is one of those recipes that look fancy with minimal effort. Chalk it up to the mix of wild mushrooms seasoned well with all-purpose seasoning folded into hearty wild rice. How about serving this during winter holiday meals? It's sure to be a hit.

❧ ❧ ❧ ❧ ❧ ❧ ❧ ❧ ❧

1 cup uncooked packaged wild and white rice blend
2 tablespoons olive oil
3 garlic cloves, minced
1 medium-size onion, chopped
1 pound mixed wild mushrooms, stemmed and chopped coarsely
1 tablespoon salt-free all-purpose seasoning
¼ cup minced fresh parsley

1. Prepare the wild rice and white rice mixture according to the package directions, omitting the salt and the seasoning packet.

2. Meanwhile, heat the olive oil in a large skillet over medium heat. Add the garlic and onion and sauté for 7 to 8 minutes. Add the mushrooms, raise the heat to medium-high, and sauté, occasionally turning the mushrooms, for about 5 minutes. Add the all-purpose seasoning and continue to cook for 1 to 2 minutes.

3. Combine the cooked wild and white rice blend with the mushroom mixture and mix well. Garnish with minced parsley.

BASIC NUTRITIONAL VALUES

Calories 110
  Calories from Fat 35
Total Fat 4.0 g
  Saturated Fat 0 g
  Trans Fat 0 g
Cholesterol 0 mg
Sodium 5 mg
Total Carbohydrate 17 g
  Dietary Fiber 2 g
  Sugars 1 g
Protein 3 g

Couscous Salad

11 SERVINGS/SERVING SIZE: ½ CUP

PREPARATION TIME: 15 MINUTES

COOK TIME: 5 MINUTES

COOLING TIME: 2 HOURS

Sometimes one fresh herb can carry the flavor for the whole dish. Fresh mint is one of those herbs. The cooling sensation on your taste buds is enough to create fantastic flavor. Mint and lemon are natural partners and in this refreshing couscous salad they make a great summer side salad.

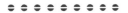

2   cups low-sodium vegetable stock
1   cup uncooked couscous
1   cup seeded and diced tomato
½   cup seeded and diced cucumber
½   cup chopped fresh mint leaves
2   scallions, minced
3   tablespoons olive oil
1   tablespoon freshly squeezed lemon juice
½   tablespoon red wine vinegar
    Freshly ground white pepper

1. Bring the vegetable stock to a boil in a small saucepan. Add the couscous, turn off the heat, cover, and let stand for 5 to 10 minutes. Fluff the couscous with a fork and transfer to a bowl. Let cool completely.

2. Add the remaining ingredients to the couscous, cover, and refrigerate for 1 hour. Bring to room temperature to serve.

BASIC NUTRITIONAL VALUES

Calories 100
  Calories from Fat 35
Total Fat 4.0 g
  Saturated Fat 0.5 g
  Trans Fat 0 g
Cholesterol 0 mg
Sodium 30 mg
Total Carbohydrate 14 g
  Dietary Fiber 1 g
  Sugars 1 g
Protein 2 g

Fennel and Orange Salad

8 SERVINGS/SERVING SIZE: ½ CUP

TIME: 30 MINUTES

COOK TIME: 0

I have dozens of clients who were self-proclaimed fennel haters until I made this salad for them! Yes, sometimes fennel can taste a bit like strong licorice, so you have to tame its wildness with something sweet, such as an orange. The honey in the dressing also brings out fennel's softer side. A dash of all-purpose seasoning finishes the dressing nicely.

❧ ❧ ❧ ❧ ❧ ❧ ❧ ❧

1 medium-size fennel bulb
2 large oranges, peeled and sectioned
½ medium-size red onion, sliced thinly
4 cups bite-size pieces of romaine lettuce

Dressing
2 tablespoons freshly squeezed lemon juice
1 tablespoon honey
1 teaspoon salt-free all-purpose seasoning
1 teaspoon Dijon mustard
1 garlic clove, minced finely
¼ cup olive oil

1. Chop off the top, base, and tough outer parts of the fennel. Cut the bulb into very thin slices.

2. Combine the fennel, oranges, red onion, and lettuce in a large bowl.

3. In a small bowl, whisk together the lemon juice, honey, all-purpose seasoning, mustard, and garlic. Slowly, in a thin stream, whisk in the oil until the dressing is emulsified. Drizzle the dressing over the salad. Let sit for 10 minutes so that the flavors mingle. Serve the salad in individual bowls or on plates.

BASIC NUTRITIONAL VALUES

Calories 110
  Calories from Fat 65
Total Fat 7.0 g
  Saturated Fat 1.0 g
  Trans Fat 0 g
Cholesterol 0 mg
Sodium 35 mg
Total Carbohydrate 12 g
  Dietary Fiber 3 g
  Sugars 8 g
Protein 1 g

Steak Fries

8 SERVINGS/SERVING SIZE: 2 PIECES

PREPARATION TIME: 6 MINUTES

COOK TIME: 40 MINUTES

You can keep shoestring fries; I like mine with some heft to them! This four-ingredient recipe is all you need to create a substantial side dish. You won't miss the salt; the all-purpose seasoning, coupled with paprika and cracked black pepper, spices up basic potatoes quite well.

❋ ❋ ❋ ❋ ❋ ❋ ❋ ❋ ❋

2 tablespoons canola oil
1 tablespoon salt-free all-purpose seasoning
½ teaspoon paprika
¼ teaspoon cracked black pepper
2 large baking potatoes, washed

1. Preheat the oven to 400°F. Line a baking sheet with parchment paper.

2. In a bowl, combine the oil, all-purpose seasoning, paprika, and black pepper. Mix well.

3. Cut each potato into quarters lengthwise and then cut each quarter in half crosswise to form wedges. Add the potatoes to the oil mixture. Mix well to coat the potatoes with the seasonings.

4. Arrange the potatoes on the prepared baking sheet in one layer without overcrowding the pan. Bake the potatoes for about 15 minutes. Turn the wedges over and bake for another 15 minutes, until well browned.

BASIC NUTRITIONAL VALUES

Calories 105
  Calories from Fat 30
Total Fat 3.5 g
  Saturated Fat 0 g
  Trans Fat 0 g
Cholesterol 0 mg
Sodium 10 mg
Total Carbohydrate 16 g
  Dietary Fiber 2 g
  Sugars 1 g
Protein 2 g

Lemon Pepper Brussels Sprouts with Pancetta

9 SERVINGS/SERVING SIZE: ½ CUP

PREPARATION TIME: 10 MINUTES

COOK TIME: 30 MINUTES

As far as I am concerned, the only way to prepare Brussels sprouts is to roast them. I remember the days when all I knew how to do was to boil them. Needless to say, everyone sort of picked around the sprouts. Now, by roasting them with Lemon Pepper seasoning and garnishing them with some crispy pancetta, the lowly sprouts deserve a place at any dinner table.

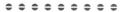

1 pound Brussels sprouts, trimmed and halved
2 tablespoons olive oil
1 to 2 teaspoons salt-free Lemon Pepper seasoning
1 ounce pancetta (about 2 slices)
1 small onion, diced
1 garlic clove, minced
1 tablespoon freshly squeezed lemon juice

1. Preheat the oven to 400°F. Line a baking sheet with parchment paper. In a bowl, combine the Brussels sprouts with 1 tablespoon of the olive oil and the Lemon Pepper seasoning. Toss well. Place the Brussels sprouts on the prepared baking sheet in a single layer.

2. Roast the sprouts for 20 to 25 minutes, until cooked through and crispy.

3. Meanwhile, heat the remaining tablespoon of olive oil. Add the pancetta and sauté until the pancetta is crispy. Remove the pancetta from the skillet and set aside to cool. Add the onion and garlic to the skillet and sauté over medium heat for 5 to 6 minutes, until the onion is soft. Crumble the pancetta into small pieces and add to the onion mixture.

4. Toss the cooked Brussels sprouts with the lemon juice in a bowl. Top with the onion mixture.

BASIC NUTRITIONAL VALUES

Calories 60
　Calories from Fat 40
Total Fat 4.5 g
　Saturated Fat 1.0 g
　Trans Fat 0 g
Cholesterol 5 mg
Sodium 70 mg
Total Carbohydrate 5 g
　Dietary Fiber 2 g
　Sugars 1 g
Protein 2 g

Southwestern Coleslaw

10 SERVINGS/SERVING SIZE: 1 CUP

TIME: 30 MINUTES

COOK TIME: 0

This salad's zippy flavor comes from adding salt-free Southwest Chipotle seasoning. It makes the humble cabbage a flavorful alternative to traditional mayonnaise- and sodium-laden slaw.

● ● ● ● ● ● ● ● ●

7 cups shredded green cabbage
3 medium-size carrots, peeled and grated
1 small red bell pepper, seeded, cored, and diced
3 scallions, minced
1 small jalapeño pepper, minced

Dressing
¼ cup apple cider vinegar
1 tablespoon freshly squeezed lime juice
1 tablespoon honey
1 to 2 teaspoons salt-free Southwest Chipotle seasoning
⅓ cup olive oil

Garnish
¾ cup pecan pieces

1. Combine the cabbage, carrots, red bell pepper, scallions, and jalapeño pepper in a large salad bowl and toss well.

2. In a small bowl, whisk together the cider vinegar, lime juice, honey, and Southwest Chipotle seasoning. Slowly, in a thin stream, add the olive oil, whisking constantly until the salad dressing is emulsified. Add the dressing to the coleslaw and mix well.

3. Toast the pecan pieces in a 6-inch dry skillet over medium heat until lightly browned, shaking the pan occasionally. Watch carefully so the nuts do not burn. Transfer the toasted pecans to a bowl. Garnish the salad with toasted pecans.

DID YOU KNOW?

Unlike spices, sodium does not offer any healthful compounds such as antioxidants or flavonoids.

BASIC NUTRITIONAL VALUES

Calories 155
  Calories from Fat 125
Total Fat 14.0 g
  Saturated Fat 1.5 g
  Trans Fat 0 g
Cholesterol 0 mg
Sodium 25 mg
Total Carbohydrate 9 g
  Dietary Fiber 3 g
  Sugars 5 g
Protein 2 g

Chopped Vegetable Salad with Garlic Herb Dressing

6 SERVINGS/SERVING SIZE: 1 CUP

PREPARATION TIME: 15 MINUTES

COOK TIME: 0

Always serving a tossed green salad? Go off the beaten track with a rich mix of crunchy vegetables instead. A fresh lemon, garlic, and herb dressing makes these vegetables anything but boring. You can use the dressing for marinating meat, poultry, or seafood as well.

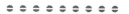

1 large English cucumber, peeled, seeded, and chopped
½ large red bell pepper, cored, seeded, and diced
½ yellow bell pepper, cored, seeded, and diced
1 cup chopped cherry tomatoes
3 scallions, minced

Dressing

2 tablespoons freshly squeezed lemon juice
1 to 2 teaspoons salt-free Garlic & Herb seasoning
¼ teaspoon Dijon mustard
Pinch of sugar
3 tablespoons olive oil

Fresh spinach leaves, washed gently and patted dry

1. In a large salad bowl, combine the cucumber, red and yellow bell pepper, cherry tomatoes, and scallions.

2. In a small bowl, whisk together the lemon juice, Garlic & Herb seasoning, mustard, and sugar. Slowly, in a thin stream, whisk in the olive oil until the dressing is emulsified. Add the dressing to the vegetables. Serve over the spinach leaves.

BASIC NUTRITIONAL VALUES

Calories 85
    Calories from Fat 65
Total Fat 7.0 g
    Saturated Fat 1.0 g
    Trans Fat 0 g
Cholesterol 0 mg
Sodium 10 mg
Total Carbohydrate 5 g
    Dietary Fiber 1 g
    Sugars 3 g
Protein 1 g

Eggplant Stuffed with Cilantro Pesto

8 SERVINGS/SERVING SIZE: 1

PREPARATION TIME: 20 MINUTES

COOK TIME: 10 MINUTES

This is two recipes in one. Instead of the usual basil pesto, why not try a more assertive cilantro one instead? This bold pesto is stuffed into baked eggplant slices and is a welcome change from ho-hum side dishes.

❧ ❧ ❧ ❧ ❧ ❧ ❧ ❧

BASIC NUTRITIONAL VALUES

Calories 210
  Calories from Fat 180
Total Fat 20.0 g
  Saturated Fat 3.0 g
  Trans Fat 0 g
Cholesterol 5 mg
Sodium 25 mg
Total Carbohydrate 8 g
  Dietary Fiber 3 g
  Sugars 3 g
Protein 3 g

1 large eggplant
Cooking spray
½ cup olive oil
½ cup walnuts
2½ cups coarsely chopped fresh cilantro
1 garlic clove, minced
Juice and zest of ½ lemon
¼ cup freshly grated Parmesan cheese

1. Preheat the oven to 425°F. Coat two baking sheets with cooking spray.

2. Slice the eggplant lengthwise into eight ½-inch slices.

3. Distribute the eggplant slices between the baking sheets. Brush each slice generously with 2 teaspoons of the olive oil. Bake for 10 minutes, until lightly browned. When done, let the eggplant cool on the sheets.

4. Toast the walnuts in a 6-inch dry skillet over medium heat until lightly browned, shaking the pan occasionally. Watch carefully so the nuts do not burn. Transfer the toasted walnuts to a bowl.

5. Place the cilantro, walnuts, garlic, lemon juice, and lemon zest in a food processor. Slowly add the remaining olive oil, processing until the pesto is smooth (add additional olive oil if needed). Add the Parmesan cheese and process for 10 seconds.

6. Place 1 tablespoon of pesto at the widest end of each eggplant slice and roll up. If there is extra pesto, save for another use in a covered container and use within 2 days.

Haricots Verts with Cherry Tomatoes

4 SERVINGS/SERVING SIZE: ½ CUP

PREPARATION TIME: 5 MINUTES

COOK TIME: 13 MINUTES

Side dishes are more often than not an afterthought. But with side dishes such as these crunchy bright green beans and sweet cherry tomatoes, you might think of this before you plan the main dish! A slice of Italy is present in this basil-laced dish that's so easy to prepare, you'll pair it with so many others.

❂ ❂ ❂ ❂ ❂ ❂ ❂ ❂

1 tablespoon olive oil
1 large shallot, sliced thinly
1 teaspoon salt-free Italian seasoning
8 ounces trimmed haricot verts green beans
¼ cup low-sodium, reduced-fat chicken stock (page 123)
½ cup halved grape tomatoes
Juice of ½ lemon
5 large fresh basil leaves, sliced thinly

1. Heat the oil in a large skillet over medium heat. Add the shallot and sauté for 3 minutes. Add the Italian seasoning and sauté for 1 minute.

2. Add the beans and with tongs turn them to coat with the shallots. Add the stock, cover, and steam for 4 minutes, until the beans turn bright green but are still crisp. Add the grape tomatoes, cover, and steam for 1 minute. Uncover and continue to cook until the grape tomatoes are just beginning to soften, about 2 minutes.

3. Add the lemon juice and basil and serve.

BASIC NUTRITIONAL VALUES

Calories 60
  Calories from Fat 30
Total Fat 3.5 g
  Saturated Fat 0.5 g
  Trans Fat 0 g
Cholesterol 0 mg
Sodium 10 mg
Total Carbohydrate 7 g
  Dietary Fiber 2 g
  Sugars 2 g
Protein 2 g

Perfect Corn on the Cob

6 SERVINGS/SERVING SIZE: 1 EAR CORN

PREPARATION TIME: 5 MINUTES

COOK TIME: 6 MINUTES

Skip the pats of butter on corn on the cob in favor of these creative oil spreads. Here are two recipes for infusing olive oil with sprightly Lemon Pepper and golden-hued tandoori-style spice.

＊＊＊＊＊＊＊＊

6 large ears corn

Lemon Pepper Oil

½ cup olive oil

1 tablespoon finely minced scallion (white part only)

1 teaspoon salt-free Lemon Pepper seasoning

or

Curry Oil

½ cup olive oil

1 tablespoon grated fresh lime zest

½ teaspoon salt-free tandoori-style seasoning

1. Husk and remove the silk from the ears of corn. Place the corn in a large pot and add just enough water to cover. Bring to a boil, then boil for 2 minutes. Drain.

2. Coat the grill rack on an outdoor grill with high-heat cooking spray. Heat the grill to medium-high. Choose a flavored oil and combine all its ingredients. Brush the oil over each ear of corn. Place the corn on the grill and grill for 3 to 4 minutes just until grill marks appear.

BASIC NUTRITIONAL VALUES

Calories 275

    Calories from Fat 180

Total Fat 20.0 g

    Saturated Fat 2.5 g

    Trans Fat 0 g

Cholesterol 0 mg

Sodium 0 mg

Total Carbohydrate 25 g

    Dietary Fiber 3 g

    Sugars 5 g

Protein 4 g

Herbes de Provence Squash

8 SERVINGS/SERVING SIZE: ½ SQUASH

PREPARATION TIME: 10 MINUTES

COOK TIME: 10 MINUTES

I was first introduced to herbes de Provence, well, when I was in Provence! Little beautiful jars of the tantalizing mixture lined just about every little shop from Arles to Aix en Provence. I just love having some around whether I end up cooking with it or not. Inhaling the aroma of the herbs, with its hint of lavender, always brings me back to happy days in sunny France.

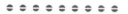

2 medium-size zucchini
2 medium-size yellow squash
1 tablespoon minced garlic
⅓ cup olive oil
1 teaspoon herbes de Provence
  Pinch of crushed red
  pepper flakes

Garnish
Fresh lemon wedges

1. Slice the zucchini and yellow squash lengthwise into long, ⅓-inch-thick slices. Place the slices in a single layer on two large baking pans.

HERBES DE PROVENCE

Herbes de Provence is a mix of dry herbs typical of the Provence region in Southeast France. The mix of herbs varies widely and usually includes basil, fennel seed, lavender, oregano, rosemary, tarragon, and thyme. Although it traditionally is a blend of dried herbs, fresh herbs can also be used.

2. Place the garlic and oil in a small saucepan and cook over medium-low heat for 6 to 7 minutes, just until fragrant. Add the herbes de Provence.

3. Pour the oil mixture evenly over all the zucchini and yellow squash and let stand for 10 minutes.

4. Prepare an outdoor grill. Coat the grill rack with cooking spray. Heat the grill to medium-high. Carefully place the zucchini and yellow squash on the grill, arranging them so the slices do not fall through the grill rack. Cook the squash until browned, 4 to 6 minutes per side. Serve the squash with lemon wedges.

BASIC NUTRITIONAL VALUES

Calories 95
  Calories from Fat 80
Total Fat 9.0 g
  Saturated Fat 1.5 g
  Trans Fat 0 g
Cholesterol 0 mg
Sodium 5 mg
Total Carbohydrate 4 g
  Dietary Fiber 1 g
  Sugars 2 g
Protein 1 g

Grilled Italian Plum Tomatoes

4 SERVINGS/SERVING SIZE: 1 PLUM
TOMATO

TIME: 10 MINUTES

COOK TIME: 10 MINUTES

Take tomatoes to a new level by grilling them! As delicate as plum tomatoes seem, they really do hold their teardrop shape when cooked at grilling temperatures. And you'll find those who are usually eager to add some salt won't even ask where the shaker is.

● ● ● ● ● ● ● ●

1   tablespoon minced garlic
¼   cup olive oil
1 to 2   teaspoons salt-free Italian seasoning
4   large plum tomatoes, halved lengthwise

Garnish
2   teaspoons freshly grated Parmesan cheese

1. In a small skillet, combine the garlic and oil. Heat over medium-low heat for 6 to 7 minutes, just until fragrant and the garlic is just beginning to brown. Add the Italian seasoning.

2. Place the tomatoes cut side up on a baking pan. Brush the cut side of the tomatoes with some of the garlic oil.

3. Prepare an outdoor grill. Transfer the tomatoes to the grill, cut side down, and brush additional garlic oil on top (skin side) of the tomatoes. Grill the tomatoes for 3 to 5 minutes per side, or until grill marks appear and the tomatoes soften. Serve the tomatoes cut side up, garnished with Parmesan cheese.

BASIC NUTRITIONAL VALUES

Calories 145
  Calories from Fat 125
Total Fat 14.0 g
  Saturated Fat 2.0 g
  Trans Fat 0 g
Cholesterol 0 mg
Sodium 15 mg
Total Carbohydrate 4 g
  Dietary Fiber 1 g
  Sugars 2 g
Protein 1 g

Kale Salad with Currants

6 SERVINGS/SERVING SIZE: ½ CUP

PREPARATION TIME: 15 MINUTES

COOK TIME: 0

I must give kudos to the fabulous restaurant Posana, located in Asheville, North Carolina, for inspiring this salad. The restaurant prepares a fabulous kale salad that I couldn't get enough of when I was there a year ago. While I didn't ask for the recipe, I just kept drawing on the tastes I remembered so fondly. The flavors are all so perfectly balanced with the sweetness from the currants and the richness from the pine nuts and cheese. The Lemon Pepper seasoning gives it a lingering fresh taste.

⊜ ⊜ ⊜ ⊜ ⊜ ⊜ ⊜ ⊜

BASIC NUTRITIONAL VALUES

Calories 205
  Calories from Fat 135
Total Fat 15.0 g
  Saturated Fat 1.5 g
  Trans Fat 0 g
Cholesterol 0 mg
Sodium 30 mg
Total Carbohydrate 17 g
  Dietary Fiber 2 g
  Sugars 10 g
Protein 4 g

⅓ cup pine nuts
3 cups washed, dried, and finely chopped fresh kale leaves, inner rib removed and discarded
½ cup dried currants
¼ cup very finely minced shallot

Dressing
2 tablespoons freshly squeezed lemon juice
1 tablespoon champagne vinegar
1 teaspoon salt-free Lemon Pepper seasoning
1 garlic clove, minced finely
1 teaspoon sugar
¼ cup walnut oil

Garnish
1 teaspoon shaved Manchego cheese per serving

1. Toast the pine nuts in a 6-inch dry skillet over medium heat until lightly browned, shaking the pan occasionally. Watch carefully so the nuts do not burn. Transfer the toasted pine nuts to a bowl.

2. Combine the kale, currants, toasted pine nuts, and shallots in a large bowl.

3. In a small bowl, whisk together the lemon juice, champagne vinegar, Lemon Pepper seasoning, garlic, and sugar. Slowly, in a thin stream, whisk in the oil until the dressing is emulsified.

4. Add the dressing to the kale and toss well, using tongs.

5. Serve the kale salad on individual plates and top with Manchego cheese.

Israeli Couscous "Tabbouleh" Salad

16 SERVINGS/SERVING SIZE: ½ CUP

PREPARATION TIME: 35 MINUTES

COOK TIME: 18 MINUTES

To tell the truth, I never really cared for traditional tabbouleh salad. I'm just not a big fan of bulgur wheat, I suppose, but I do love the parsley, tomatoes, and lemon juice dressing. When I began using Israeli couscous several years ago, I thought, why not replace the bulgur with the couscous, and a new version of tabbouleh was born.

● ● ● ● ● ● ● ● ●

2 teaspoons olive oil
1 cup Israeli couscous
1¼ cups water
1½ cups minced fresh flat-leaf parsley
½ cup minced fresh mint
3 large tomatoes, cubed
2 scallions, sliced

Dressing
3 tablespoons freshly squeezed lemon juice
1 teaspoon salt-free Lemon Pepper seasoning
⅓ cup olive oil

1. Heat the 2 teaspoons of oil in a large skillet over medium heat. Add the couscous and toast for about 3 minutes. Add the water and bring to a boil. Cover the skillet, lower the heat to a simmer, and cook until the water is absorbed, about 15 minutes. Transfer the couscous to a bowl and let cool.

2. Add the parsley, mint, tomatoes, and scallions to the couscous.

3. Whisk together the lemon juice, Lemon Pepper seasoning, and ⅓ cup of olive oil. Add to the couscous and toss well. Cover and refrigerate for 30 minutes to meld the flavors.

BASIC NUTRITIONAL VALUES
Calories 90
  Calories from Fat 45
Total Fat 5.0 g
  Saturated Fat 0.5 g
  Trans Fat 0 g
Cholesterol 0 mg
Sodium 10 mg
Total Carbohydrate 10 g
  Dietary Fiber 1 g
  Sugars 1 g
Protein 2 g

Italian Black Rice Salad

11 SERVINGS/SERVING SIZE: ½ CUP

PREPARATION TIME: 10 MINUTES (RICE DOES NEED TO SOAK OVERNIGHT)

COOK TIME: 35 MINUTES

Ever try black rice? It's such an incredible backdrop color for bright, crunchy vegetables. Unanimously my testers described this salad as "gorgeous"! You'll never miss salt in this dish; the dressing hits all tastes on the palate just right.

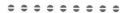

1   cup uncooked black rice
1¾ cups water
2   large tomatoes, seeded and cut into small cubes
1   medium-size yellow bell pepper, cored, seeded, and diced
2   scallions, minced
1   celery stalk, chopped
10 fresh basil leaves, chopped

Dressing
3   tablespoons red wine vinegar
1   tablespoon freshly squeezed lemon juice
1   garlic clove, minced
1   teaspoon salt-free Italian seasoning
½   teaspoon sugar
¼   cup olive oil

Garnish
Almond slivers or pine nuts (optional)

1. Soak the rice overnight in a large bowl of water to cover. Drain very well through a fine sieve.

2. Bring the 1¾ cups of water to a boil in a large saucepan. Add the soaked rice and bring to a boil. Lower the heat, cover, and simmer for 35 minutes, until tender.

3. Turn the rice out of the saucepan into a large bowl and let cool.

4. Meanwhile, prepare the dressing: In a small bowl, whisk together the vinegar, lemon juice, garlic, Italian seasoning, and sugar. Slowly, in a thin stream, whisk in the oil until the dressing is emulsified. Set aside.

5. When the rice has cooled, add the tomatoes, yellow bell pepper, scallions, celery, and basil to the rice. Mix well. Add about half of the dressing and mix again.

6. Toast the almonds or pine nuts in a 6-inch dry skillet over medium heat until lightly browned, shaking the pan occasionally. Watch carefully so the nuts do not burn. Transfer the nuts to a bowl. Garnish the salad with toasted almonds or pine nuts. Serve with additional dressing on the side.

BASIC NUTRITIONAL VALUES

Calories 120
    Calories from Fat 55
Total Fat 6.0 g
    Saturated Fat 1.0 g
    Trans Fat 0 g
Cholesterol 0 mg
Sodium 10 mg
Total Carbohydrate 16 g
    Dietary Fiber 1 g
    Sugars 2 g
Protein 2 g

Butternut Squash and Chickpea Salad

8 SERVINGS/SERVING SIZE: ½ CUP

PREPARATION TIME: 20 MINUTES

COOK TIME: 15 MINUTES

I first learned of this combination of ingredients from a most unlikely source: the Sydney, Australia, airport! While waiting for a flight connection, I had the most scrumptious salad of butternut squash (they call it pumpkin) tossed with chickpeas and raisins in a fresh, slightly spicy lemon juice dressing. If this is airport food, well, I'll take it anytime. Here's my version of that wonderful memory.

❂ ❂ ❂ ❂ ❂ ❂ ❂ ❂

1 small butternut squash
1 large carrot, peeled and diced
1 large celery stalk, diced
3 scallions, white part only, minced
1 (15-ounce) can no-salt-added chickpeas, drained and rinsed
½ cup golden raisins

Dressing
3 tablespoons freshly squeezed lemon juice
1½ teaspoons salt-free Southwest Chipotle seasoning
½ teaspoon Dijon mustard
½ teaspoon sugar
⅓ cup olive oil

Garnish
¼ cup roasted unsalted cashews

1. Peel, seed, and cut the butternut squash into ½-inch cubes. Place the squash in a large saucepan. Cover with water and bring to a boil. Cook the squash over medium-high heat just until tender, about 15 minutes. Drain the squash and let cool for 30 minutes.

2. In a large bowl, combine the squash with the carrot, celery, scallions, chickpeas, and raisins.

3. In a small bowl, whisk together the lemon juice, Southwest Chipotle seasoning, mustard, and sugar. In a thin stream, slowly add the olive oil and whisk until the dressing is emulsified. Add the dressing to the squash salad and toss gently. Garnish the salad with the cashews.

BASIC NUTRITIONAL VALUES

Calories 220
  Calories from Fat 110
Total Fat 12.0 g
  Saturated Fat 2.0 g
  Trans Fat 0 g
Cholesterol 0 mg
Sodium 30 mg
Total Carbohydrate 26 g
  Dietary Fiber 5 g
  Sugars 9 g
Protein 5 g

Beet, Carrot, and Daikon Salad with Ginger Five-Spice Dressing

11 SERVINGS/SERVING SIZE: ½ CUP

PREPARATION TIME: 5 MINUTES

COOK TIME: 0

I always like to include a recipe in my cookbooks that makes you feel as if you are a star chef. This salad is so visually stunning, it rivals anything served in an upscale restaurant. I love the piquant dressing. It's also great over steamed green beans or broccoli.

⊜ ⊜ ⊜ ⊜ ⊜ ⊜ ⊜ ⊜ ⊜ ⊜

BASIC NUTRITIONAL VALUES

Calories 70
  Calories from Fat 55
Total Fat 6.0 g
  Saturated Fat 0.5 g
  Trans Fat 0 g
Cholesterol 0 mg
Sodium 25 mg
Total Carbohydrate 5 g
  Dietary Fiber 1 g
  Sugars 3 g
Protein 1 g

2 medium-size beets, peeled
2 medium-size carrots, peeled
1 medium-size daikon radish, peeled

Dressing
2 tablespoons rice vinegar
2 tablespoons freshly squeezed lime juice
2 teaspoons peeled and minced fresh ginger
1 garlic clove, minced
2 teaspoons toasted sesame oil
1½ teaspoons sugar
1 teaspoon Chinese five-spice powder
3 tablespoons canola oil

Garnish
2 tablespoons white or black sesame seeds

1. Using a food processor or handheld grater, coarsely shred the beets, carrots, and daikon separately. Place the piles of beets, carrots, and daikon side by side on a platter.

> **CHINESE FIVE-SPICE POWDER**
> Chinese five-spice powder is a mixture of five spices commonly used in China and other Asian countries. Although the proportion of ingredients varies, the mixture often includes star anise, cloves, cinnamon, fennel, and Sichuan pepper. The fragrant mixture is often used to flavor pork and duck.

2. In a small bowl, whisk together the rice vinegar, lime juice, ginger, garlic, sesame oil, sugar, and Chinese five-spice powder. Slowly, in a thin stream, whisk in the canola oil until the dressing is emulsified.

3. Drizzle the salad dressing over the piles of beets, carrots, and daikon.

4. Toast the sesame seeds in a 6-inch dry skillet over medium heat until lightly browned, shaking the pan occasionally. Watch carefully so the seeds do not burn. Transfer the toasted seeds to a bowl. Sprinkle toasted sesame seeds over all.

Simply Roasted Garlic Asparagus

7 SERVINGS/SERVING SIZE: 5 SPEARS

PREPARATION TIME: 15 MINUTES

COOK TIME: 10 TO 12 MINUTES

Sometimes cooking vegetables is just that simple. Got a pan, an oven, and about twelve minutes to spare? Roasting is a perfect technique to achieve golden brown asparagus spears with a slight crunch. All asparagus need is a touch of garlic and herbs and it becomes a staple side dish.

❧ ❧ ❧ ❧ ❧ ❧ ❧ ❧

1   pound medium-width asparagus
1   teaspoon salt-free Garlic & Herb seasoning
1½ tablespoons olive oil

1. Preheat the oven to 425°F. Line a baking sheet with parchment paper.

2. Break off the tough ends of the asparagus. Lightly peel the bottoms of the stalks. Arrange the asparagus in a single layer on the prepared baking sheet.

3. Whisk the Garlic & Herb seasoning into the olive oil. Brush the olive oil mixture over the asparagus and roast for 10 to 12 minutes, until tender.

BASIC NUTRITIONAL VALUES

Calories 35
  Calories from Fat 25
Total Fat 3.0 g
  Saturated Fat 0 g
  Trans Fat 0 g
Cholesterol 0 mg
Sodium 0 mg
Total Carbohydrate 1 g
  Dietary Fiber 1 g
  Sugars 0 g
Protein 1 g

Braised Root Vegetables with Garam Masala

4 SERVINGS/SERVING SIZE: 1 CUP

PREPARATION TIME: 20 MINUTES

COOK TIME: 1 HOUR AND 10 MINUTES

Braising vegetables is a technique that is often overlooked. I think it sounds so much more intimidating than it really is. In this recipe, root vegetables are simply sautéed with bold seasonings of cumin and garam masala and then left to simmer in a bath of orange juice and broth. The result is a warm pot of inviting flavors.

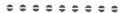

3 tablespoons olive oil

2 teaspoons ground cumin

1 teaspoon garam masala ••••••••••

6 large shallots, peeled and halved

2 large carrots, peeled and cut into 2-inch chunks

2 large parsnips, peeled and cut into 2-inch chunks

1 small sweet potato, peeled and cut into 2-inch chunks

1 cup peeled and cubed turnip

1½ cups low-sodium, reduced-fat chicken stock (page 123)

¼ cup freshly squeezed orange juice

½ cup diced dried apricots

2 teaspoons honey

¼ teaspoon freshly ground black pepper

GARAM MASALA
Garam masala literally means "hot mixture." *Hot* refers to the intensity and warming properties of the spices, rather than denoting a spicy or fiery flavor. In India, the spice blend in garam masala will vary from family to family and can include bay leaves, black pepper, cardamom, cinnamon, coriander, cloves, cumin, ginger, nutmeg, mustard seeds, and many other spices.

Garnish

¼ cup finely minced fresh parsley

1. Heat the oil in a large Dutch oven over medium heat. Add the cumin and garam masala and heat for 1 minute.

2. Add the shallots and sauté for 3 minutes. Add the carrots, parsnips, sweet potato, and turnip and sauté for 8 to 10 minutes, until browned.

3. Add the stock and orange juice. Transfer the pan to the oven and bake for 45 to 50 minutes, until the vegetables are very tender. During the last 10 minutes of cooking, mix in the apricots.

4. Drizzle in the honey and grind in the black pepper and mix well. Garnish with minced parsley.

Caribbean Sweet Potatoes

6 SERVINGS/SERVING SIZE: ½ CUP

PREPARATION TIME: 10 MINUTES

COOK TIME: 40 MINUTES

This recipe requires little preparation, but the outcome looks complex. This mashed sweet potato dish is a nice spicy-sweet alternative to brown sugar—drowned or worse, marshmallow-topped sweet potatoes!

❖ ❖ ❖ ❖ ❖ ❖ ❖ ❖

3 medium-size sweet potatoes
2 tablespoons orange juice concentrate
1 tablespoon brown sugar
2 teaspoons salt-free Caribbean Citrus seasoning
1 teaspoon unsalted butter
¼ teaspoon ground ginger

1. Preheat the oven to 400°F. Prick the skin of the sweet potatoes all over with a fork. Place the sweet potatoes directly on the oven rack and place a foil-lined baking sheet on the rack below the sweet potatoes to catch any juices. Bake the sweet potatoes for about 45 minutes to 1 hour, or until the sweet potatoes are tender.

2. Remove the sweet potatoes from the oven and let cool for 5 to 10 minutes. Scoop out the sweet potato pulp and discard the skins. Transfer the sweet potatoes to a large bowl. Add the remaining ingredients and mash well with a potato masher to the desired consistency.

BASIC NUTRITIONAL VALUES

Calories 75
  Calories from Fat 10
Total Fat 1.0 g
  Saturated Fat 0 g
  Trans Fat 0 g
Cholesterol 0 mg
Sodium 30 mg
Total Carbohydrate 17 g
  Dietary Fiber 2 g
  Sugars 8 g
Protein 1 g

Watercress and Radicchio Salad

8 SERVINGS/SERVING SIZE: 1 CUP

PREPARATION TIME: 20 MINUTES

COOK TIME: 0

Watercress gets it due in this gorgeous salad. The visual pop of the red tomatoes and purple radicchio nestled among vibrant greens of the salad makes for an impressive presentation.

❋ ❋ ❋ ❋ ❋ ❋ ❋ ❋ ❋

BASIC NUTRITIONAL VALUES

Calories 100
  Calories from Fat 80
Total Fat 9.0 g
  Saturated Fat 1.0 g
  Trans Fat 0 g
Cholesterol 0 mg
Sodium 10 mg
Total Carbohydrate 4 g
  Dietary Fiber 1 g
  Sugars 2 g
Protein 1 g

1 bunch fresh watercress, washed and patted dry, tough stems removed
1 small head romaine lettuce, washed and patted dry, torn into bite-size pieces
1 cup shredded radicchio
1 cup halved grape tomatoes
½ small red onion, sliced very thinly

Lemon thyme dressing
3 tablespoons red wine vinegar
1 tablespoon freshly squeezed lemon juice
1 tablespoon minced fresh lemon thyme
1 small garlic clove, minced
1 teaspoon sugar
¼ cup walnut oil
  Freshly ground black pepper

Garnish
¼ cup chopped walnuts

1. Mix together the watercress, romaine, radicchio, grape tomatoes, and red onion in a large bowl. Toss well.

2. For the dressing, whisk together the red wine vinegar, lemon juice, lemon thyme, garlic, and sugar. Slowly, in a thin stream, whisk in the walnut oil until the salad dressing is emulsified. Season with freshly ground black pepper to taste.

3. Toast the walnuts in a 6-inch dry skillet over medium heat until lightly browned, shaking the pan occasionally. Watch carefully so the nuts do not burn. Transfer the toasted walnuts to a bowl.

4. Arrange the salad on individual plates. Drizzle with the dressing and garnish with toasted walnuts.

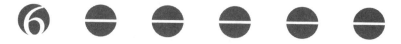

Soups

CHICKEN STOCK THREE WAYS

Here are three different recipes to make great-tasting chicken stock that is low in sodium. The recipes start with the one with the longest cooking time and then move to the one with the shortest cooking time. Depending on what ingredients you have on hand and your time constraint, choose one of these three ways to make perfectly delicious and versatile chicken stock.

The first recipe features wings, backs, and bone-in thighs, as they produce the richest-tasting broth. The simmering time is the longest—over two hours. When you have the time, this is the recipe I'd encourage you to make, as it is rich, deep, and flavorful.

You'll find the second chicken stock recipe described in the Old-Fashioned Chicken and Rice Soup recipe on page 134. In this recipe, the preparation is similar to this first one; however, chicken parts are called for, though not necessarily necks and backs. It's a bit lighter in flavor and the simmering time is shorter.

As for the third recipe, if all you have on hand is canned or boxed stock, make sure it's the lowest in sodium you can find. The stock will most likely taste bland, so here is a way to zip up the flavor: For every quart of chicken stock, add ½ pound of chicken wings; 1 large carrot, cut into chunks; ½ large onion, chopped coarsely; 1 celery stalk, chopped coarsely; and 2 whole black peppercorns. Bring the entire mixture to a boil in a large saucepan, lower the heat, partially cover, and simmer for 30 minutes, strain, and use in your favorite recipes.

Use any of these three recipes when chicken stock is called for throughout this chapter and in other chapters in this book.

Homemade Chicken Stock

MAKES 3½ QUARTS OR 12
SERVINGS/SERVING SIZE: 1 CUP

PREPARATION TIME: 5 MINUTES PLUS 1
HOUR TO SOAK

COOK TIME: 2–3 HOURS AND 15
MINUTES

3 pounds combination of chicken backs, wings, and bone-in thighs
2 large yellow onions, chopped coarsely, skins left on
2 large carrots, cut into chunks
1 celery stalk, cut into chunks
1 sprig fresh thyme
1 bay leaf
½ lemon
3 whole peppercorns
3½ quarts cold water

1. Place the chicken wings and backs in a large bowl with water to cover. This will help release any excess blood and create a clearer broth. Soak the chicken for about 1 hour.

2. Drain the water from the chicken parts and rinse. Place the chicken parts in a large, heavy stockpot.

3. Add the remaining ingredients to the pot and bring to a boil. Lower the heat, partially cover, and simmer for 2–3 hours. Skim occasionally to remove impurities from the broth.

4. Strain the broth through a fine sieve; the best tool to use for this is a conical strainer called a chinois. Press out all the liquid from the solid ingredients. Taste the broth and adjust the seasoning.

5. Refrigerate the stock overnight so that the fat has a chance to rise to the top and solidify. Remove the fat and discard. Place the chicken stock in quart containers, label, and freeze for up to 3 months. To use, defrost the stock in the refrigerator and reheat.

BAY LEAVES

Bay leaves are the leaves of the bay laurel tree. In ancient Greece, the leaves of the laurel tree were considered a symbol of victory and success. Victorious Olympic athletes would be crowned with a headpiece made of bay leaves. The term *laureate* comes from this ancient practice of being distinguished in a particular field with a laurel (bay leaf) wreath.

BASIC NUTRITIONAL VALUES

Calories 15
    Calories from Fat 0
Total Fat 0.0 g
    Saturated Fat 0 g
    Trans Fat 0 g
Cholesterol 5 mg
Sodium 10 mg
Total Carbohydrate 1 g
    Dietary Fiber 0 g
    Sugars 1 g
Protein 1 g

Italian Roasted Red Pepper Soup with Garlic Croutons

6 SERVINGS/SERVING SIZE: 1¼ CUPS

PREPARATION TIME: 20 MINUTES

COOK TIME: 1 HOUR AND 10 MINUTES

Roasted red peppers are the perfect antidote to the salt shaker habit. Their natural sweetness counteracts any need for a salty soup. Flecks of the Italian seasoning are so attractive in this warming soup. This soup can be made a day ahead or frozen up to the point before adding the milk and cream. Thaw in the refrigerator overnight and place in a saucepan to heat through. Add the milk and cream. The croutons may also be made one or two days in advance.

☙ ☙ ☙ ☙ ☙ ☙ ☙ ☙

BASIC NUTRITIONAL VALUES

Calories 230
  Calories from Fat 90
Total Fat 10.0 g
  Saturated Fat 3.0 g
  Trans Fat 0 g
Cholesterol 15 mg
Sodium 155 mg
Total Carbohydrate 29 g
  Dietary Fiber 4 g
  Sugars 13 g
Protein 7 g

Roasted Peppers and Onions

2 teaspoons olive oil
4 large red bell peppers
2 large onions, peeled, halved, and sliced into ½-inch pieces

Soup

1 cup Homemade Chicken Stock (page 123)
1 tablespoon olive oil
2 garlic cloves, minced
2 teaspoons salt-free Italian seasoning
2 cups 1% milk
½ cup light cream
  Freshly ground black pepper

Croutons

4 (½-inch) slices French bread
1 tablespoon olive oil
1 teaspoon salt-free Garlic & Herb seasoning

1. Preheat the oven to 425°F. Coat a baking sheet with 1 teaspoon of the oil. Halve and seed the bell peppers. Arrange them cut side down on the prepared baking sheet.

2. Toss the remaining teaspoon of olive oil with the onions. Spread the onions on another baking sheet in a single layer. Place the tray of peppers on the oven's upper rack and the onions on the lower rack. Roast the peppers for about 40 minutes and the onions for about 30 minutes. Stir the onions occasionally.

3. Remove the vegetables from the oven and let cool. Peel off and discard the pepper skins.

4. Transfer the peppers and onions to a food processor or blender and process until smooth. Add 2 tablespoons of the chicken stock or water if necessary to make the mixture smooth.

5. Heat the 1 tablespoon of olive oil in a large saucepan. Add the garlic and sauté over medium-low heat for 2 minutes. Add the Italian seasoning and sauté for 1 minute. Add the pepper puree, milk, and stock. Bring to a simmer and simmer over low heat for 10 minutes. Add the cream and simmer 1 minute. Season with freshly ground black pepper.

6. To prepare the croutons: Brush each piece of French bread with olive oil. Cut each slice into ½-inch cubes. Sprinkle each cube with the Garlic & Herb seasoning. Bake for 4 to 6 minutes at 400°F, until lightly toasted.

Indian Lentil Soup

4 SERVINGS/SERVING SIZE: 1¼ CUPS

PREPARATION TIME: 12 MINUTES

COOK TIME: 45 MINUTES

Lentils (and most beans, for that matter) usually require some sodium to bring out their flavor—unless you know how to use spices instead. Tandoori is one of the best seasoning blends to use to draw out the natural earthiness of everyone's favorite little lentil. The cool, ginger-infused yogurt topping is the perfect foil for this slightly spicy soup.

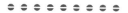

1 tablespoon olive oil
1 large onion, chopped
3 garlic cloves, minced
2 teaspoons salt-free tandoori-style seasoning
1 (14.5-ounce) can no-salt-added diced tomatoes
2½ cups water
½ cup dried brown lentils, picked over and rinsed

Topping
½ cup plain low-fat yogurt
1 teaspoon peeled, grated fresh ginger
1 teaspoon freshly squeezed lemon juice
½ teaspoon sugar

1. Heat the olive oil in a large saucepan over medium heat. Add the onion and garlic and sauté for 6 to 8 minutes, until the onion is golden. Add the tandoori-style seasoning and sauté for 1 minute.

2. Add the tomatoes with their juice, and the water and lentils. Bring to a boil, lower the heat, cover, and simmer over low heat for about 30 minutes, until the lentils are tender.

3. For the topping, combine the yogurt, ginger, lemon juice, and sugar. Add a dollop of the yogurt mixture to each bowl of soup.

BASIC NUTRITIONAL VALUES

Calories 175
  Calories from Fat 40
Total Fat 4.5 g
  Saturated Fat 1.0 g
  Trans Fat 0 g
Cholesterol 0 mg
Sodium 70 mg
Total Carbohydrate 27 g
  Dietary Fiber 7 g
  Sugars 9 g
Protein 9 g

Southwestern Two-Bean Chili

5 SERVINGS/SERVING SIZE: 1 CUP

PREPARATION TIME: 5 MINUTES

COOK TIME: 35 MINUTES

Dinner in about 30 minutes or less? Absolutely, thanks to the pantry staples in this easy recipe. The Southwest Chipotle seasoning makes the beans sparkle with a rich taste, more than salt could possibly do.

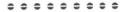

2	tablespoons olive oil
1	large onion, chopped
1	tablespoon salt-free Southwest Chipotle seasoning
1	(14.5-ounce) can no-salt-added diced tomatoes
1	tablespoon chili sauce
2	cups low-sodium, reduced-fat chicken stock (page 123)
1	(15-ounce) can no-salt-added red kidney beans, drained and rinsed
1	(15-ounce) can no-salt-added black beans, drained and rinsed
1	cup frozen corn

Sour cream topping

½	cup reduced-fat sour cream
1	teaspoon salt-free Southwest Chipotle seasoning

1. Heat the oil in a large saucepan over medium-high heat. Add the onion and sauté for 3 minutes. Add the tablespoon of Southwest Chipotle seasoning and sauté for 2 minutes.

> **DID YOU KNOW?**
> A 30- to 45-second rinse under cold running tap water reduces the sodium content of canned beans by about 35 percent.

2. Add the tomatoes with their juice, and the chili sauce and stock and bring to a boil. Lower the heat and simmer for 10 minutes. Add the beans and simmer for 10 minutes. Add the corn and simmer for 5 minutes.

3. Combine the sour cream and the teaspoon of Southwest Chipotle seasoning. Top each bowl of chili with a dollop and serve.

BASIC NUTRITIONAL VALUES

Calories 285
  Calories from Fat 70
Total Fat 8.0 g
  Saturated Fat 2.5 g
  Trans Fat 0 g
Cholesterol 10 mg
Sodium 145 mg
Total Carbohydrate 41 g
  Dietary Fiber 10 g
  Sugars 9 g
Protein 14 g

Zuppa di Ceci

6 SERVINGS/SERVING SIZE: 1 CUP

PREPARATION TIME: 10 MINUTES

COOK TIME: 40 MINUTES

I've learned so many wonderful soups on my trips to Tuscany. This one is by far my favorite. I still have glorious memories of picking fresh rosemary, basil, and sage out of the kitchen garden. One of the best moments was when one of my teachers wryly admonished Americans for using too much salt. She simply said, "When you learn how to properly use fresh and dried herbs and spices, you'll never miss the salt."

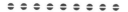

BASIC NUTRITIONAL VALUES

Calories 290
    Calories from Fat 70
Total Fat 8.0 g
    Saturated Fat 1.0 g
    Trans Fat 0 g
Cholesterol 0 mg
Sodium 150 mg
Total Carbohydrate 46 g
    Dietary Fiber 10 g
    Sugars 10 g
Protein 12 g

2 tablespoons olive oil
1 large celery stalk, chopped finely
1 large onion, chopped finely
1 small sprig fresh rosemary, chopped finely
6 sage leaves, chopped finely
4 garlic cloves, minced finely
1 (28-ounce) can no-salt-added whole tomatoes
2 (15-ounce) cans no-salt-added chickpeas, drained and rinsed
4 tablespoons finely chopped fresh basil
¼ teaspoon freshly ground black pepper
1 tablespoon freshly squeezed lemon juice

Garnish

6 slices Italian bread (⅔ ounce per slice)
2 to 3 garlic cloves, halved lengthwise

1. Heat the olive oil in a large saucepan over medium heat. Add the celery, onion, rosemary, and sage and sauté for about 8 minutes. Add the garlic and sauté for 2 minutes.

2. Place the tomatoes in a large bowl. With your hands, crush the tomatoes, leaving them slightly coarse. Add the tomatoes with their juices to the pan.

3. Puree one can of the chickpeas in a food processor or blender with ¼ cup of water until smooth but still thick. Add the pureed chickpeas and the other can of whole chickpeas to the soup. Add the basil and black pepper and bring the soup to a boil. Lower the heat and simmer for 15 minutes.

4. Add the lemon juice. Correct the consistency of the soup by adding water if necessary.

5. Just before serving, toast the Italian bread slices. Once the bread is toasted, rub one side of the bread with the garlic. Top each bowl of soup with a slice of garlic toast.

Lemon Asparagus Soup

8 SERVINGS/SERVING SIZE: 1 CUP

PREPARATION TIME: 10 MINUTES

COOK TIME: 40 MINUTES

When my recipe tester tasted this soup she said it reminded her of dining at a decadent gourmet restaurant. But little does she know that this soup's humble beginnings came from whatever my mom had on hand. Asparagus was always a favorite vegetable in our home, and when it was in season my mom always made this flavorful soup. I guess my mom was a salt-free pioneer; she never added salt to soups and always favored Lemon Pepper seasoning instead.

● ● ● ● ● ● ● ● ●

BASIC NUTRITIONAL VALUES

Calories 160

Calories from Fat 90

Total Fat 10.0 g

Saturated Fat 4.0 g

Trans Fat 0 g

Cholesterol 25 mg

Sodium 25 mg

Total Carbohydrate 16 g

Dietary Fiber 3 g

Sugars 3 g

Protein 5 g

1 tablespoon olive oil
1 small leek, bottom portion only, washed and chopped
1 medium-size onion, chopped
2 garlic cloves, minced
2 pounds asparagus, stems trimmed, sliced into 2-inch pieces
2 large russet potatoes, peeled and cubed
6 cups Homemade Chicken Stock (page 123)
1 tablespoon salt-free Lemon Pepper seasoning
½ cup heavy cream

Garnishes
¼ cup chopped pistachio nuts
Freshly grated zest of 1 lemon

1. Heat the olive oil in a large saucepan over medium heat. Add the leek, onion, and garlic and sauté for 7 to 9 minutes, until vegetables are soft. Add the asparagus, potatoes, and stock. Bring to a boil, lower the heat to medium, and cook until the potatoes are tender, 15 to 17 minutes.

2. Ladle the soup into a food processor or blender and process until the soup is smooth, working in batches if necessary. Return the soup to the saucepan and add the Lemon Pepper seasoning and cream. Heat through for 1 minute.

3. Toast the pistachios in a 6-inch dry skillet over medium heat until lightly browned, shaking the pan occasionally. Watch carefully so the nuts do not burn. Transfer the toasted pistachios to a bowl.

4. Garnish each bowl with lemon zest and pistachio nuts.

Shrimp Bisque

8 SERVINGS/SERVING SIZE: 1 CUP

PREPARATION TIME: 30 TO 35 MINUTES

COOK TIME: 60 MINUTES

Making your own shrimp broth is easy and replaces the need for the high-sodium chicken stock usually called for in bisques. The Lemon Pepper seasoning brightens and folds beautifully into this seaside-flavored soup.

❧ ❧ ❧ ❧ ❧ ❧ ❧ ❧

2 pounds shell-on shrimp
1 tablespoon unsalted butter
2 medium-size onions, diced
2 medium-size carrots, peeled and diced
2 medium-size celery stalks, diced
1 tablespoon tomato paste
2 teaspoons salt-free Lemon Pepper seasoning
2 medium-size bay leaves
¼ teaspoon crushed red pepper flakes
½ teaspoon minced fresh tarragon
5 cups water
¼ cup all-purpose flour
¼ cup plus 2 tablespoons dry sherry
⅔ cup 1% milk
¼ cup half-and-half

1. Peel the shrimp and reserve the shells. Devein the shrimp and then coarsely chop them into bite-size pieces, about 1 inch long. Place in a container and keep refrigerated until ready to use.

2. Melt the butter in a 5-quart pot over medium-high heat. Add the onions, carrots, celery, and reserved shrimp shells. Cook until the shells are pink and slightly tender, 5 to 8 minutes.

3. Add the tomato paste, Lemon Pepper seasoning, bay leaves, crushed red pepper flakes, and tarragon and cook for 1 minute. Add the water and bring to a boil. Lower the heat to low and simmer uncovered for about 45 minutes, until the broth has acquired the flavor of the shrimp shells and aromatics. Strain through a fine sieve, set aside the liquid, and discard the solids.

4. Mix together the flour and sherry and whisk until smooth. Return the shrimp broth to the pot and slowly add the sherry mixture, whisking constantly. Bring to a boil. Lower the heat to medium and add the milk, half-and-half, and one-quarter of the reserved chopped shrimp. Cook for 7 to 8 minutes over medium heat.

5. Remove the pot from the heat. Place the remaining shrimp and 1 cup of the broth in a food processor or blender and process until the mixture is smooth (or blend well with an immersion blender). Add the pureed mixture back to the pot. Heat for 1 minute and serve.

BASIC NUTRITIONAL VALUES

Calories 120
    Calories from Fat 30
Total Fat 3.5 g
    Saturated Fat 2.0 g
    Trans Fat 0 g
Cholesterol 130 mg
Sodium 195 mg
Total Carbohydrate 6 g
    Dietary Fiber 0 g
    Sugars 2 g
Protein 15 g

Cool Gazpacho

7 SERVINGS/SERVING SIZE: 1 CUP

PREPARATION TIME: 15 MINUTES

COOK TIME: 0

I'm always puzzled why anyone would add salt to gazpacho. It has so much flavor from fresh vegetables, lime juice, and a zip of hot sauce. The addition of salt-free all-purpose seasoning adds just the right amount of herb flavor and completes this refreshing, clean-tasting summer soup.

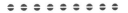

3 cups no-salt-added tomato juice

1 cup low-sodium, reduced-fat chicken stock (page 123)

1 large tomato, seeded and chopped

1 medium-size green bell pepper, cored, seeded, and diced

1 small cucumber, peeled, seeded, and diced

2 scallions, minced

2 tablespoons red wine vinegar

1 tablespoon freshly squeezed lime juice

1 tablespoon olive oil

1 tablespoon salt-free all-purpose seasoning
  Hot sauce
  Freshly ground black pepper

1. Combine all the ingredients in a large bowl, adding hot sauce and freshly ground pepper to taste. Refrigerate for 3 to 4 hours.

2. Puree half of the gazpacho in a food processor or blender until smooth. Add back to the remaining gazpacho and serve chilled.

BASIC NUTRITIONAL VALUES

Calories 55
  Calories from Fat 20
Total Fat 2.0 g
  Saturated Fat 0 g
  Trans Fat 0 g
Cholesterol 0 mg
Sodium 90 mg
Total Carbohydrate 8 g
  Dietary Fiber 1 g
  Sugars 5 g
Protein 2 g

Thai Shrimp Soup

7 SERVINGS/SERVING SIZE: 1 CUP

PREPARATION TIME: 15 MINUTES

COOK TIME: 25 MINUTES

When you think of Asian soups, soy sauce and other salty ingredients are often standard. But they are not always necessary. In this soup, fresh lemongrass along with lime zest, pungent cilantro, and hot peppers give this soup its wow factor.

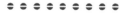

6 cups Homemade Chicken Stock (page 123)
3 stalks fresh lemongrass, lower part only, sliced diagonally into three pieces, crushed slightly
  Zest of 1 lime
1 small serrano pepper, seeded and diced
1 pound large peeled and deveined shrimp, tails removed
2 tablespoons freshly squeezed lime juice

Garnishes
4 scallions, white part only, minced
¼ cup minced fresh cilantro
1 small red Thai chili pepper, minced

1. Place the stock, lemongrass, and lime zest in a large saucepot over high heat. Bring to a boil, lower the heat, cover, and simmer for 20 minutes.

2. Strain the broth and return it to the saucepot. Add the pepper and shrimp and simmer over low heat for 3 to 5 minutes, until the shrimp are just cooked through. Stir in the lime juice.

3. Garnish each bowl with scallions, cilantro, and chili pepper.

BASIC NUTRITIONAL VALUES

Calories 70
  Calories from Fat 10
Total Fat 1.0 g
  Saturated Fat 0 g
  Trans Fat 0 g
Cholesterol 95 mg
Sodium 115 mg
Total Carbohydrate 4 g
  Dietary Fiber 0 g
  Sugars 1 g
Protein 11 g

Cucumber Soup

3 SERVINGS/SERVING SIZE: 1 CUP

PREPARATION TIME: 15 MINUTES

COOK TIME: 0

Sprinkling salt over cucumber can ruin the natural sweet taste. This creamy soup proves all you need is a handful of really fresh herbs to make cucumbers shine.

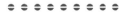

4 small cucumbers, peeled, seeded, and grated
1½ cups plain fat-free Greek yogurt
½ cup crème fraîche
2 teaspoons fresh lemon zest
2 tablespoons freshly squeezed lemon juice
½ cup chopped fresh mint
½ cup chopped fresh dill
1 tablespoon olive oil
¼ teaspoon ground white pepper

Garnishes

2 tablespoons minced fresh dill
½ cup fresh cooked, cold baby shrimp

1. Place all the ingredients except the garnishes in a food processor or blender. Puree until smooth. Pour the soup into a container and refrigerate for 3 to 4 hours to meld the flavors. Garnish the soup with chopped dill and baby shrimp. Excellent served with a slice of whole-grain rye bread!

DILL

Dill is very fragile, in both its fresh and dry forms, and should not be boiled as the leaves will lose their flavor. It is preferable to add dill leaves after a dish has been cooked, so as to retain their flavor and aroma. After harvesting, dill has a tendency to wilt very quickly. Wrap it in a paper towel and store in a re-sealable plastic bag to extend its freshness. Dill can also be frozen.

BASIC NUTRITIONAL VALUES

Calories 290
  Calories from Fat 170
Total Fat 19.0 g
  Saturated Fat 10.0 g
  Trans Fat 0 g
Cholesterol 100 mg
Sodium 125 mg
Total Carbohydrate 12 g
  Dietary Fiber 2 g
  Sugars 8 g
Protein 18 g

Southwestern Squash and Leek Soup

10 SERVINGS/SERVING SIZE: 1 CUP

PREPARATION TIME: 20 MINUTES

COOK TIME: 1 HOUR AND 15 MINUTES

Usually squash soups have a sweet bent. I thought it would be more intriguing to go off the beaten path and make this soup spicy instead. It has a fun kick and attractive swirls of yogurt and crème fraîche, for a different version of the typical autumn soup.

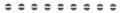

BASIC NUTRITIONAL VALUES

Calories 120
  Calories from Fat 65
Total Fat 7.0 g
  Saturated Fat 3.0 g
  Trans Fat 0 g
Cholesterol 15 mg
Sodium 20 mg
Total Carbohydrate 12 g
  Dietary Fiber 3 g
  Sugars 3 g
Protein 3 g

1 large butternut squash
2 tablespoons olive oil
2 cups chopped, well-washed leeks, white part only (about 2 medium-size leeks)
½ tablespoon salt-free Southwest Chipotle seasoning
¼ cup dry white wine
4 ½ cups Homemade Chicken Stock (page 123)
1 teaspoon ground white pepper
1 tablespoon unsalted butter

Topping

3 tablespoons pumpkin seeds
½ cup plain nonfat yogurt
¼ cup crème fraîche
1 tablespoon minced fresh chives

1. To make it easier to cut the squash, microwave the butternut squash on high for 5 to 6 minutes. Remove the squash carefully with pot holders and set aside until cool enough to handle. If you do not have a microwave oven or you wish to skip this step, proceed with step 2.

2. Cut the squash in half crosswise. Standing each piece upright, carefully peel the skin off each piece with a sharp knife or sharp vegetable peeler. Discard the skin. Set each piece of squash lengthwise on a cutting board. Cut each piece in half lengthwise. Remove and discard the seeds from the bottom half of the squash. Using a serrated spoon, remove any excess fibers that are stringy from the bottom half of the squash. Cut all the squash into 1-inch cubes.

3. Heat the olive oil over medium heat in a large saucepan. Add the squash and leeks and sauté for 5 minutes. Add the Southwest Chipotle seasoning and sauté for 2 minutes. Add the wine and stock. Cover and bring to a boil over medium-high heat. Lower the heat to a simmer and cook until the squash is tender, about 25 minutes. Let cool for 15 minutes.

4. Add the white pepper. Puree the soup, in batches if necessary, in a food processor or blender (or use an immersion blender). Add the soup back to the saucepot and add the butter. Heat over low heat for a few minutes, just until the butter melts.

5. For the topping, toast the pumpkin seeds in a small, dry skillet for 2 to 3 minutes, shaking the pan frequently, until lightly browned. Set aside. In a small bowl, combine the yogurt, crème fraîche, and chives. For each bowl of soup, swirl the yogurt mixture on top. Garnish with pumpkin seeds.

Old-Fashioned Chicken and Rice Soup

14 SERVINGS/SERVING SIZE: 1 CUP

PREPARATION TIME: 10 MINUTES

COOK TIME: 3 HOURS

CHILLING TIME: OVERNIGHT

Ever look at the sodium content of most canned or boxed chicken soups? Let's just say the numbers are truly astounding. But not here. Everyone loves a good chicken soup when a bit under the weather. This soup, made with fresh herbs, is sure to resolve all your ills.

⊜ ⊜ ⊜ ⊜ ⊜ ⊜ ⊜ ⊜

Chicken Stock

1 (4-pound) chicken, cut into parts, washed
2 large onions, unpeeled, quartered
4 medium-size carrots, unpeeled, cut into chunks
4 large celery stalks, chopped coarsely
6 sprigs fresh parsley
6 black peppercorns
3 bay leaves

Soup

2 teaspoons olive oil
1 large onion, chopped
2 large carrots, peeled and sliced diagonally into ½-inch pieces
1 large celery stalk, sliced diagonally into ½-inch pieces
1 tablespoon salt-free all-purpose seasoning
1 cup long-grain basmati rice
Freshly ground black pepper
2 tablespoons minced fresh parsley
2 teaspoons minced fresh thyme

> **DID YOU KNOW?**
> The average can of soup contains half a day's worth of sodium!

BASIC NUTRITIONAL VALUES

Calories 130
  Calories from Fat 25
Total Fat 3.0 g
  Saturated Fat 1.0 g
  Trans Fat 0 g
Cholesterol 30 mg
Sodium 45 mg
Total Carbohydrate 14 g
  Dietary Fiber 1 g
  Sugars 2 g
Protein 11 g

1. Prepare the stock: Put the chicken parts in a heavy stockpot. Add the onions, carrots, and celery stalks. Add 3 quarts of water and bring to a boil. Skim the surface and remove any gray residue.

2. Add the parsley, peppercorns, and bay leaves. Partially cover the pan and simmer over low heat for 2 to 2½ hours. Remove the chicken parts and set aside to cool, then refrigerate overnight.

3. Line a large colander with cheesecloth and strain the broth, pressing on the solids. Discard the vegetables and reserve all the broth. Transfer the stock to a large container and refrigerate overnight.

4. Remove the stock from the refrigerator. Spoon off any solidified fat and discard; the stock should be clear.

5. Prepare the soup: In a large pot, heat the olive oil. Add the onion and sauté for 5 minutes. Add the carrots, celery, and all-purpose seasoning and sauté for 3 minutes. Add the rice and continue to cook for 2 minutes. Add the stock and bring to a boil. Lower the heat and simmer for 6 to 7 minutes.

6. While the rice is cooking, remove and discard all the bones and skin from the chicken parts. Cut about 1 pound of the chicken meat into small pieces for the soup. Save any remaining chicken for another use. Wrap the leftover chicken in an airtight container and keep in the refrigerator for up to 3 days.

7. Stir the cooked chicken into the soup and cook for 3 minutes. Season with freshly ground black pepper to taste. Sprinkle the soup with the parsley and thyme.

Moroccan Bean and Vegetable Soup with Farro

21 SERVINGS/SERVING SIZE: 1 CUP

PREPARATION TIME: 25 TO 30 MINUTES

COOK TIME: 1 HOUR AND 20 MINUTES

Ever try farro? It may sound new to you, but it's been around since ancient Rome! This high-fiber, plump grain is what makes this hearty, bean-filled soup a meal all on its own. Farro can be found in the grain section of natural food stores and many supermarkets. The tandoori-style seasoning gives this soup a beautiful flaxen color. This soup makes a huge quantity, so freeze half to enjoy at another time.

● ● ● ● ● ● ● ● ●

BASIC NUTRITIONAL VALUES

Calories 115
  Calories from Fat 25
Total Fat 3.0 g
  Saturated Fat 0 g
  Trans Fat 0 g
Cholesterol 0 mg
Sodium 30 mg
Total Carbohydrate 21 g
  Dietary Fiber 4 g
  Sugars 4 g
Protein 4 g

3 tablespoons olive oil
4 cups sliced onions (2 large onions)
2 garlic cloves, minced
1½ tablespoons salt-free tandoori-style seasoning
¼ teaspoons cayenne pepper
2 quarts Homemade Chicken Stock (page 123)
3 cups peeled and thinly sliced carrots (about 5 large carrots)
2 cups sliced zucchini (about 1 large or 2 medium-size)
2 cups sliced yellow squash (about 1 large or 2 medium-size)
4 cups peeled, thinly sliced russet potatoes (4 medium-size potatoes)
¼ cup freshly squeezed lemon juice
½ cup chopped fresh cilantro
1 (14.5-ounce) can no-salt-added chickpeas, drained and rinsed
1 (14.5-ounce) can diced no-salt-added tomatoes
1 cup uncooked farro, cooked according to the package directions, eliminating the salt (makes about 2 cups cooked farro)

1. Heat the oil in a 5-quart saucepan over medium-high heat. Add the onion and garlic and sauté for 3 minutes. Add the tandoori-style seasoning and cayenne and cook for 1 minute. Add the stock, carrots, zucchini, yellow squash, and potatoes and bring to a boil. Lower the heat and simmer, covered, for 1 hour.

2. Remove the pan from the heat and add the lemon juice and cilantro. Transfer in batches to a food processor or blender (or use an immersion blender) and puree until smooth. Return the pureed soup to a saucepan and add the chickpeas, tomatoes, and cooked farro. Simmer for 2 minutes.

Chinese Five-Spice Melon Soup

8 SERVINGS/SERVING SIZE: 1 CUP

PREPARATION TIME: 20 MINUTES

CHILLING TIME: 2 HOURS

What to do with a bumper crop of cantaloupe? Puree it into this luscious, silken, chilled soup. The trio of Chinese five-spice powder, grated ginger, and fresh Thai basil will wake up your taste buds for the next course.

❀ ❀ ❀ ❀ ❀ ❀ ❀ ❀ ❀

2 medium-size cantaloupes, peeled, seeded, and cubed
3 tablespoons heavy cream
2 tablespoons brown sugar
2 teaspoons freshly squeezed lemon juice
1 teaspoon Chinese five-spice powder
2 tablespoons grated fresh ginger
1 tablespoon sliced fresh Thai basil

1. In a food processor or blender, puree the cantaloupe with the cream, sugar, lemon juice, and Chinese five-spice powder. Transfer the puree to a pitcher.

2. Place the grated ginger in a piece of cheesecloth. Squeeze the ginger of its juice and add the juice to the cantaloupe mixture. Discard the ginger solids.

3. Cover and refrigerate the cantaloupe soup for 1 to 2 hours.

4. Pour the soup into individual bowls and garnish with the Thai basil.

BASIC NUTRITIONAL VALUES

Calories 80
　Calories from Fat 20
Total Fat 2.5 g
　Saturated Fat 1.5 g
　Trans Fat 0 g
Cholesterol 10 mg
Sodium 25 mg
Total Carbohydrate 15 g
　Dietary Fiber 1 g
　Sugars 14 g
Protein 1 g

Vidalia Onion Soup

8 SERVINGS/SERVING SIZE: 1 CUP

PREPARATION TIME: 20 MINUTES

COOK TIME: 40 MINUTES

The first onion soup I was taught to make was French onion soup. I remember slaving away getting the onions perfectly caramelized. While classic French onion soup is certainly worth the time and effort, I love onion-based soups so much that I developed this quicker method with the same rich and flavorful results. This is a creamy onion soup rather than brothy, and the sweetness of the Vidalia onion more than carries the flavor.

❊ ❊ ❊ ❊ ❊ ❊ ❊ ❊

BASIC NUTRITIONAL VALUES

Calories 130
  Calories from Fat 55
Total Fat 6.0 g
  Saturated Fat 3.5 g
  Trans Fat 0 g
Cholesterol 20 mg
Sodium 30 mg
Total Carbohydrate 15 g
  Dietary Fiber 2 g
  Sugars 8 g
Protein 3 g

2 tablespoons unsalted butter
3 large Vidalia onions (or other sweet onion), halved and sliced thinly (about 6 cups)
1 tablespoon salt-free all-purpose seasoning
1 cup white wine
6 cups Homemade Chicken Stock (page 123)
3 tablespoons all-purpose flour
¾ cup half-and-half
¼ teaspoon white pepper
1 teaspoon sugar

Garnish
½ cup minced fresh parsley

1. Melt the butter in a large saucepan over medium heat. Add the onions and cook over medium-low heat for 10 to 12 minutes, until tender; do not brown. Add the all-purpose seasoning and cook for 1 minute.

2. Add the wine and cook for 5 minutes. Add the stock and bring to a boil. Lower the heat to low and simmer for 10 minutes.

3. Whisk together the flour and half-and-half and add to the onion mixture, whisking constantly to prevent any lumps from forming. Continue heating just until tiny bubbles form around the edge of the saucepan and the broth has thickened slightly. Remove from the heat and season with white pepper and sugar. Garnish each individual bowl with parsley.

Veal and Mushroom Stew

12 SERVINGS/SERVING SIZE: 1 CUP

PREPARATION TIME: 20 MINUTES

COOK TIME: 2 HOURS AND 20 MINUTES

The first veal recipes I learned to make were mostly breaded veal and salt-laden sauces. Not exactly healthy. A better way to present veal is in stews such as this. No need for salt to carry the dish, as rich cremini mushrooms, creamy russet potatoes, bright orange carrots, tender peas, savory onions, and garlic are all enveloped in an Italian seasoning base. This is where veal belongs.

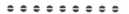

2	tablespoons all-purpose flour
3	tablespoons salt-free Italian seasoning
3	tablespoons olive oil
2	pounds veal top round, cut into ¾-inch cubes
1½	pounds cremini mushrooms, cleaned, stemmed, and quartered
4	cups Homemade Chicken Stock (page 123)
1	large onion, chopped coarsely
3	garlic cloves, minced
2	large russet potatoes, peeled and cut into ¾-inch pieces
3	medium-size carrots, peeled and sliced into ½-inch pieces
1	cup frozen peas
1	tablespoon minced fresh thyme
¼ to ½	teaspoon freshly ground black pepper

1. Combine the flour with the Italian seasoning. Heat the oil in a large Dutch oven over medium heat. Dredge the veal cubes lightly in the flour mixture and add the veal, in batches to keep the veal in one layer. Cook, turning, until well browned on each side, about 5 minutes total.

2. Remove the veal from the pan and deglaze the pan with ¼ cup of the chicken stock. Add the mushrooms and sauté for about 4 minutes, until well browned. Remove the mushrooms from the pan and deglaze with another ¼ cup of the stock. Add the onions and garlic and sauté for 4 minutes. Return the veal to the pot, add the remaining 3½ cups of stock, and bring to a boil. Partially cover, lower the heat to a simmer, and cook for 45 minutes, stirring occasionally.

3. Add the potatoes and carrots to the stew and continue to cook for another 45 minutes, or until the vegetables are tender. Add the reserved mushrooms, peas, and thyme. Season with black pepper to taste.

BASIC NUTRITIONAL VALUES

Calories 190

 Calories from Fat 55

Total Fat 6.0 g

 Saturated Fat 1.0 g

 Trans Fat 0 g

Cholesterol 65 mg

Sodium 70 mg

Total Carbohydrate 15 g

 Dietary Fiber 3 g

 Sugars 4 g

Protein 19 g

Star Anise Cold Blueberry Soup

6 SERVINGS/SERVING SIZE: ½ CUP

PREPARATION TIME: 10 MINUTES

COOK TIME: 15 MINUTES

CHILLING TIME: 2 TO 3 HOURS

Whole spices are used so infrequently, and usually only in teas or marinades, that we forget they are great to use in everyday cooking. One of my very favorite whole spices is star anise. The beautiful star-shaped spice imparts sweet and warm flavor notes that pair well with fresh, plump blueberries. Pair this soup with a lovely grilled white fish for an elegant summer meal.

❄ ❄ ❄ ❄ ❄ ❄ ❄ ❄

1½ pints fresh blueberries, washed
½ cup sugar
1 star anise
1 cup water
1 lemon, quartered
¼ cup vodka (optional)

Garnish
½ cup plain nonfat Greek yogurt

1. Place the blueberries, sugar, star anise, and water in a medium-size saucepan. Squeeze in the juice from the lemon quarters and add the quarters to the saucepan.

2. Bring to a boil, lower the heat, and simmer for 15 minutes. Let cool completely in the saucepan.

3. Remove the lemon quarters and star anise from the blueberry mixture. Add the blueberry mixture to a food processor or blender. Process until smooth. Transfer the mixture to a large bowl, cover, and refrigerate the blueberry soup for 2 to 3 hours.

4. Prior to serving, stir in the vodka if using. Garnish each bowl with a dollop of Greek yogurt.

BASIC NUTRITIONAL VALUES

Calories 115
  Calories from Fat 0
Total Fat 0.0 g
  Saturated Fat 0 g
  Trans Fat 0 g
Cholesterol 0 mg
Sodium 10 mg
Total Carbohydrate 28 g
  Dietary Fiber 2 g
  Sugars 25 g
Protein 2 g

Cream of Leek and Potato Soup

8 SERVINGS/SERVING SIZE: 1 CUP

PREPARATION TIME: 15 MINUTES

COOK TIME: 35 MINUTES

You can make an entire meal out of leek and potato soup. The topping adds creaminess to this humble but stellar soup.

❧ ❧ ❧ ❧ ❧ ❧ ❧ ❧

2   tablespoons olive oil
2   large leeks, washed, white part only, washed and sliced thickly
1   large onion, chopped
1   tablespoon salt-free all-purpose seasoning
⅛   teaspoon crushed red pepper flakes
1   pound russet potatoes, peeled and chopped
6   cups Homemade Chicken Stock (page 123) or low- or no-sodium vegetable stock
⅓   cup reduced-fat sour cream
2   tablespoons chopped fresh chives

1. Heat the oil in a large saucepan over medium heat. Add the leeks and onion and sauté over medium-low heat for 10 minutes, until very soft but not browned. Add the all-purpose seasoning and crushed red pepper flakes and sauté for 2 minutes.

2. Add the potatoes and stir to coat with the leek mixture. Add 3 cups of the stock and bring to a boil. Lower the heat, partially cover, and simmer for 20 minutes.

3. Remove the soup from the heat. Ladle the soup into a food processor or blender and blend until very smooth.

4. Add the remaining 3 cups of stock to the saucepan. Add the leek and potato puree and simmer over low heat for 3 minutes. Remove the pot from the heat and stir in the sour cream. Ladle into bowls and top with chopped chives.

BASIC NUTRITIONAL VALUES

Calories 120
  Calories from Fat 40
Total Fat 4.5 g
  Saturated Fat 1.0 g
  Trans Fat 0 g
Cholesterol 5 mg
Sodium 25 mg
Total Carbohydrate 17 g
  Dietary Fiber 2 g
  Sugars 4 g
Protein 3 g

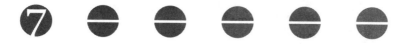

Desserts

Chocolate Chile Nut Meringues

MAKES 36 / SERVING SIZE: 3 COOKIES

PREPARATION TIME: 25 MINUTES

COOK TIME: 20 MINUTES

Savory spices in a cookie? You bet! These little meringues have a nice little kick. Spicy heat and chocolate has always been one of my favorite flavor combinations and these meringues are quite addictive.

⊜ ⊜ ⊜ ⊜ ⊜ ⊜ ⊜ ⊜ ⊜

⅓ cup coarsely chopped walnuts
½ cup plus 1 tablespoon confectioners' sugar
4 teaspoons good-quality unsweetened cocoa powder
½ teaspoon salt-free Southwest Chipotle seasoning
¼ teaspoon ground cinnamon
2 large egg whites

1. Preheat the oven to 300°F. Line two baking sheets with parchment paper. Toast the walnuts in a small skillet over medium heat until crisp and fragrant, about 6 minutes. Set aside.

2. Sift together ½ cup of the sugar, the cocoa powder, Southwest Chipotle seasoning, and cinnamon on a sheet of waxed paper.

3. Beat the egg whites with an electric beater until stiff peaks form. Very gently fold the cocoa mixture into the egg whites. Gently fold in the walnuts.

4. Drop the batter by large teaspoonfuls onto the prepared baking sheets, spacing them 1 inch apart. Bake until set, 20 to 25 minutes. Remove from the oven and let cool on a wire rack. Sprinkle with the remaining confectioners' sugar.

CINNAMON

Although there are many species of cinnamon, the two most common commercial varieties are cassia, or Chinese cinnamon, and Ceylon cinnamon. They are similar in taste, but cassia bark is thicker and has a stronger flavor. Ceylon cinnamon bark is fine and easily crumbled, more aromatic, and has a subtler flavor.

BASIC NUTRITIONAL VALUES

Calories 50
  Calories from Fat 20
Total Fat 2.5 g
  Saturated Fat 0 g
  Trans Fat 0 g
Cholesterol 0 mg
Sodium 10 mg
Total Carbohydrate 7 g
  Dietary Fiber 0 g
  Sugars 6 g
Protein 1 g

Caribbean Citrus Pineapple

6 SERVINGS/SERVING SIZE: 4 OUNCES

PREPARATION TIME: 10 MINUTES

COOK TIME: 4 MINUTES

Now you can enjoy the tropics even in the dead of the winter. Warm glazed pineapple with a surprising bit of heat and spice makes not only a nice dessert but paired with grilled seafood, chicken, or pork, an unusual side dish.

❂ ❂ ❂ ❂ ❂ ❂ ❂ ❂ ❂

1 medium-size pineapple
2 tablespoons freshly squeezed lime juice
2 teaspoons salt-free Caribbean Citrus seasoning
1 tablespoon unsalted butter
2 tablespoons brown sugar

1. Cut the leaves and stem end from the pineapple. Remove the skin and "eyes." Slice the pineapple into rings. Cut each slice into thirds and remove the hard core.

2. Place the pineapple pieces in a large bowl. Add the lime juice and Caribbean Citrus seasoning and toss well. Let stand for 20 minutes.

3. Melt the butter in a large skillet over medium heat. Add the brown sugar and heat until the sugar melts. Add the pineapple slices and cook until the pineapple is warmed through and is glazed, about 5 minutes.

BASIC NUTRITIONAL VALUES

Calories 75
  Calories from Fat 20
Total Fat 2.0 g
  Saturated Fat 1.5 g
  Trans Fat 0 g
Cholesterol 5 mg
Sodium 20 mg
Total Carbohydrate 15 g
  Dietary Fiber 1 g
  Sugars 12 g
Protein 1 g

Apple Thyme Upside-Down Cake

8 SERVINGS/SERVING SIZE: 1 SLICE

PREPARATION TIME: 15 MINUTES

COOK TIME: 42 MINUTES

Many years ago I participated in a "baking with herbs" class sponsored by a local arboretum. Our instructor, a horticulturist, gave wonderful instruction on how to add fresh herbs to baked goods, cakes, pies, and cookies. During that class I gravitated to lemon thyme as a favorite to add to treats. This cake has a rich, deep autumn focus. It's dense and moist and perfect with a warm cup of tea.

⚉ ⚉ ⚉ ⚉ ⚉ ⚉ ⚉ ⚉ ⚉

BASIC NUTRITIONAL VALUES

Calories 255
Calories from Fat 65
Total Fat 7.0 g
Saturated Fat 4.5 g
Trans Fat 0 g
Cholesterol 65 mg
Sodium 115 mg
Total Carbohydrate 44 g
Dietary Fiber 1 g
Sugars 26 g
Protein 4 g

2 tablespoons dark brown sugar
2 firm Granny Smith apples, peeled, cored, and sliced into ⅓-inch slices
1¼ cups cake flour
1 teaspoon ground cinnamon
¾ teaspoon baking powder
¼ teaspoon baking soda
¼ cup unsalted butter
¾ cup sugar
2 tablespoons minced fresh lemon thyme leaves
2 whole eggs
¾ cup low-fat buttermilk

1. Preheat the oven to 350°F. Coat a 9-inch round cake pan with cooking spray. Sprinkle the brown sugar evenly over the bottom of the pan.

2. Arrange the apples over the brown sugar in concentric circles, making sure the bottom is covered.

3. In a bowl, combine the flour, cinnamon, baking powder, and baking soda. In another bowl, beat together the butter and sugar with electric beaters. Add the thyme and eggs to the butter mixture and beat until thick.

4. Alternately fold the flour mixture and buttermilk into the egg mixture until just blended.

5. Pour the batter over the apples, smoothing the top. Bake for 35 minutes, or until a cake tester inserted comes out clean. Transfer to a cooling rack. Let the cake cool for 10 minutes in the pan. Invert the cake onto a plate and let cool slightly. Cut into slices.

Coconut Arborio Rice and Kaffir Lime Leaf Pudding

6 SERVINGS/SERVING SIZE: ½ CUP

PREPARATION TIME: 5 MINUTES

COOK TIME: 40 MINUTES

When I visited Thailand many years ago, I became totally enthralled with Kaffir lime leaves. They are typically added to Thai foods either in shredded form or whole to infuse flavor. At a cooking class in Bangkok, I added whole Kaffir lime leaves to rice as it steamed. What a wonderful aroma! I figured it might work well for rice pudding, too. So here's my Thai-inspired take on rice pudding with the subtle flavor of Kaffir lime.

❖ ❖ ❖ ❖ ❖ ❖ ❖ ❖

BASIC NUTRITIONAL VALUES

Calories 185
   Calories from Fat 45
Total Fat 5.0 g
   Saturated Fat 3.5 g
   Trans Fat 0 g
Cholesterol 5 mg
Sodium 65 mg
Total Carbohydrate 31 g
   Dietary Fiber 0 g
   Sugars 14 g
Protein 4 g

¾ cup Arborio rice
2 cups 1% milk
2 cups light coconut milk
¼ cup sugar
1 vanilla bean, split
2 fresh Kaffir lime leaves

Garnish
Ground cinnamon

1. In a large, heavy-bottomed pot, combine the rice, milk, coconut milk, sugar, and vanilla bean. Bring to a gentle boil over high heat. Lower the heat to medium and continue to cook for 30 to 40 minutes, stirring frequently to prevent the rice from sticking to the bottom of the pan and to help release the starch from the Arborio rice. The mixture should be gently boiling the entire time, but be sure it is never at a hard, rolling boil. During the last 10 minutes of cooking, add the Kaffir lime leaves. When ready, the rice should look very creamy and the rice grains should be slightly firm but cooked through.

2. If you wish to serve the rice pudding cold, stop cooking the rice pudding when it still looks a bit runny; it will firm up as it chills in the refrigerator. Remove the Kaffir lime leaves from the pudding and discard. Pour the rice pudding from the pot into a bowl. Cover the surface of the pudding with plastic wrap (this is to prevent a skin forming on the surface of the rice) and refrigerate for several hours. Proceed as below to serve.

3. If you wish to serve the rice pudding warm, remove the lime leaves from the pudding and discard. Serve the rice in individual dessert dishes. Dust the tops with cinnamon.

Berries in Ginger Peppercorn Syrup

8 SERVINGS/SERVING SIZE: 1 TABLESPOON

PREPARATION TIME: 7 MINUTES

COOK TIME: 25 MINUTES

Frankly, I think whole spices are under-utilized in cooking. Making infusions with them gives such nice flavor to so many foods. Here I just love the combination of light heat from the peppercorns and warmth from the fresh ginger slices. This zesty sauce really makes plain berries come alive. The whole mixture makes a great "adult" sauce over creamy ice cream.

● ● ● ● ● ● ● ●

1 cup dry red wine (merlot, pinot noir, Sangiovese, or light-bodied Chianti)
¼ cup sugar
12 whole black peppercorns
4 (1-inch) strips peeled fresh ginger
2 (2-inch) strips orange zest
1 whole cinnamon stick
3 cups hulled and sliced fresh strawberries
3 cups fresh raspberries, washed gently
   Scoops of light ice cream or frozen yogurt (optional)

1. Combine the wine, sugar, peppercorns, ginger, orange zest, and cinnamon stick in a small saucepan. Bring to a boil, lower the heat, and simmer for about 20 minutes, until the liquid is reduced to syrup.

2. Strain the sauce through a fine sieve with a bowl underneath. Discard the solids. Add the strawberries and raspberries to the syrup and toss gently to coat. Serve over light ice cream or frozen yogurt if desired.

BASIC NUTRITIONAL VALUES

Calories 75
  Calories from Fat 0
Total Fat 0.0 g
  Saturated Fat 0 g
  Trans Fat 0 g
Cholesterol 0 mg
Sodium 0 mg
Total Carbohydrate 17 g
  Dietary Fiber 4 g
  Sugars 12 g
Protein 1 g

Chinese Five-Spice Powder Fruit Kebabs

12 SERVINGS/SERVING SIZE: 1 SKEWER

PREPARATION TIME: 15 MINUTES

COOK TIME: 7 TO 10 MINUTES

Although grilled fruit is quite common, these kebabs are anything but. The exotic and sophisticated flavors of the fruit and spices belie their ease of preparation. Everything caramelizes so beautifully you'll think you're eating candy!

❧ ❧ ❧ ❧ ❧ ❧ ❧ ❧ ❧

BASIC NUTRITIONAL VALUES

Calories 55
  Calories from Fat 0
Total Fat 0.0 g
  Saturated Fat 0 g
  Trans Fat 0 g
Cholesterol 0 mg
Sodium 0 mg
Total Carbohydrate 14 g
  Dietary Fiber 1 g
  Sugars 12 g
Protein 0 g

Basting sauce

½ cup unsweetened pineapple juice
1 tablespoon brown sugar
  Juice of 1 lime

Fruits

1 medium-size pineapple, peeled, eyes removed, cored, and cut into 1-inch cubes
2 medium-size mangoes, peeled and cut into 1-inch cubes
2 medium-size kiwifruits, peeled and cut into 1-inch cubes
1 tablespoon Chinese five-spice powder

1. Soak twelve wooden skewers in a shallow pan with hot water to cover. Set aside for 1 hour or more.

2. Prepare an outdoor grill. Coat a grill rack with cooking spray and heat the grill to medium heat.

3. Combine all the ingredients for the basting sauce in a shallow bowl.

4. Remove the skewers from the water bath. Using two skewers for each kebab, thread the fruit, alternating the colors onto the skewers. Thread the fruit from top to bottom (this will keep the fruit flat and will prevent it from spinning on the skewer while grilling). Sprinkle the kebabs lightly with Chinese five-spice powder.

5. Place the kebabs on the grill and using a basting brush, baste the fruit with some of the basting sauce. Grill until the fruit softens and browns, 7 to 10 minutes, while lightly basting every few minutes. Be careful not to burn the fruit. Drizzle the fruit kebabs with any basting sauce that remains. Serve immediately.

Chinese Five-Spice Double Chocolate Pudding

6 SERVINGS/SERVING SIZE: ½ CUP

PREPARATION TIME: 10 MINUTES

COOK TIME: 20 MINUTES

Chocolate pudding isn't kid stuff anymore. This unexpected chocolate pudding is a sophisticated take on an old favorite. Chinese five-spice powder adds layers of flavor to the double punch of chocolate.

❁ ❁ ❁ ❁ ❁ ❁ ❁ ❁

BASIC NUTRITIONAL VALUES

Calories 305
  Calories from Fat 145
Total Fat 16.0 g
  Saturated Fat 9.0 g
  Trans Fat 0 g
Cholesterol 105 mg
Sodium 60 mg
Total Carbohydrate 39 g
  Dietary Fiber 3 g
  Sugars 32 g
Protein 7 g

6 ounces dark chocolate (bar or chips)
1 tablespoon unsalted butter
2⅓ cups low-fat 1% milk
½ cup sugar
2 tablespoons dark unsweetened cocoa powder
1 tablespoon cornstarch
1 teaspoon Chinese five-spice powder
2 egg yolks plus 1 whole egg
1 teaspoon pure vanilla extract

Garnish
Dark chocolate shavings

1. Place a large bowl in the refrigerator (this will be the bowl the pudding is stored in as it chills).

2. In a double boiler over simmering water, melt the dark chocolate and butter.

3. Meanwhile, in a large saucepot, combine 2 cups of the milk and ¼ cup of the sugar and simmer over medium-low heat. In a small bowl, mix together the cocoa, cornstarch, Chinese five-spice powder and remaining ⅓ cup of milk. Add the cocoa mixture to the simmering milk.

4. In a separate bowl, mix together the egg yolks and whole egg with the remaining ¼ cup of sugar. Whisk in some of the hot simmering milk mixture to eggs to warm them. Add the egg mixture to the saucepot. Raise the heat to medium-high and stir the pudding until thickened, about 5 minutes.

5. Whisk in the melted chocolate mixture and the vanilla and remove from the heat. Pour the pudding into the prepared chilled bowl. Cover the pudding with plastic wrap placed directly on its surface. This will prevent a skin from forming. Chill the pudding for several hours.

6. Garnish with chocolate shavings and serve.

Baked Apples with Garam Masala

6 SERVINGS/SERVING SIZE: 1 APPLE

PREPARATION TIME: 15 MINUTES

COOK TIME: 1 HOUR AND 10 MINUTES

These baked apples are a step above the predictable baked apples with cinnamon. By using garam masala, which is usually reserved for only main dishes, these apples have more layers of complex flavors. Apples are earthy fruits that can take the strong flavors present in garam masala: the spicy pepper, the sweet star anise, the warm coriander, and all the other aromatics in this classic Indian spice.

❧ ❧ ❧ ❧ ❧ ❧ ❧ ❧ ❧

BASIC NUTRITIONAL VALUES

Calories 220
  Calories from Fat 70
Total Fat 8.0 g
  Saturated Fat 3.0 g
  Trans Fat 0 g
Cholesterol 10 mg
Sodium 10 mg
Total Carbohydrate 41 g
  Dietary Fiber 6 g
  Sugars 32 g
Protein 1 g

6 large baking apples (Jonathan or McIntosh work well)
¼ cup brown sugar
¼ cup chopped walnuts
2 tablespoons unsalted butter, softened
1½ teaspoons garam masala
⅓ cup apple cider
Juice of 1 lemon

1. Preheat the oven to 350°F. With a paring knife, partially core each apple, making a well about 1 inch deep and wide. Peel the upper portion of each apple so you have about a 1-inch ring of peeled apple. Place the apples in a large baking dish.

2. In a bowl, combine the brown sugar, walnuts, butter, and garam masala. Mix well. Add a spoonful of the stuffing to the center of each apple. Pour the apple cider and the lemon juice over all the apples.

3. Bake for about 1 hour, until the apples are tender. Cover the apples at any time to prevent excessive browning if necessary.

4. Remove the apples from the baking dish and set aside. Add the pan juices to a small saucepan and reduce over medium heat for about 10 minutes, or until the juices are syrupy. Serve the apples warm or cold with the reduced pan juices spooned on top.

Blueberry Lemon Ginger Chia Seed Muffins

MAKES 12/SERVING SIZE: 1 MUFFIN

PREPARATION TIME: 30 MINUTES

COOK TIME: 23 MINUTES

These are really more like little moist baby cakes instead of having the craggy texture of traditional muffins, so they can be dessert! Chia seeds are vitamin- and mineral-packed seeds that are similar to a poppy-seed texture in baked goods. Chia seeds can be found at most natural food stores. The double ginger spice is warm and inviting.

⚫ ⚫ ⚫ ⚫ ⚫ ⚫ ⚫ ⚫ ⚫

BASIC NUTRITIONAL VALUES

Calories 195
  Calories from Fat 80
Total Fat 9.0 g
  Saturated Fat 5.0 g
  Trans Fat 0 g
Cholesterol 50 mg
Sodium 100 mg
Total Carbohydrate 24 g
  Dietary Fiber 1 g
  Sugars 12 g
Protein 4 g

½ cup unsalted butter, softened
½ cup sugar
2 large eggs
1⅓ cups all-purpose flour (use half whole wheat if desired)
3 tablespoons chia seeds
1 teaspoon baking powder
½ teaspoon baking soda
½ teaspoon ground ginger
   Zest of 2 lemons
½ cup nonfat plain Greek yogurt
1 tablespoon fat-free milk
1 tablespoon freshly squeezed lemon juice
1 teaspoon pure vanilla extract
¾ cup fresh blueberries, washed
3 tablespoons finely minced crystallized ginger

1. Preheat the oven to 350°F. Coat a twelve-cup muffin tin with cooking spray. Set aside.

2. In a large bowl, use electric beaters to cream the butter and sugar until fluffy. Add the eggs one at a time, beating well after each addition.

> ### DID YOU KNOW?
> One bakery corn muffin can have as much sodium as approximately 75 potato chips.

3. In another bowl, combine the flour, chia seeds, baking powder, baking soda, ground ginger, and lemon zest.

4. In another bowl, mix together the yogurt, milk, lemon juice, and vanilla. Add the flour and yogurt mixture alternately to the egg mixture and mix just until blended. Fold in the blueberries.

5. Divide the batter evenly among the muffin cups. Sprinkle the tops of each muffin with crystallized ginger. Bake the muffins for 20 to 25 minutes, until a toothpick inserted in the center comes out clean.

6. Remove the muffins from the oven. Let the muffins cool in the pan for 5 minutes. Run a knife around each muffin to loosen, and turn out the muffins onto a cooling rack. Let cool completely or serve warm.

Orange Macadamia Nut Bread

9 SERVINGS/SERVING SIZE: 1-INCH SLICE

PREPARATION TIME: 15 MINUTES

COOK TIME: 1 HOUR AND 5 MINUTES

The orange flavor and Chinese five-spice powder pair well in this bread. The balance of sweet and savory spices really brings out the sweet notes in the orange. And instead of the usual one-dimensional cinnamon or nutmeg in a baked good, Chinese five-spice powder elevates your cakes to a new and exciting level.

❀ ❀ ❀ ❀ ❀ ❀ ❀ ❀ ❀

BASIC NUTRITIONAL VALUES

Calories 370
Calories from Fat 135
Total Fat 15.0 g
Saturated Fat 2.0 g
Trans Fat 0 g
Cholesterol 20 mg
Sodium 170 mg
Total Carbohydrate 54 g
Dietary Fiber 2 g
Sugars 20 g
Protein 6 g

3 cups all-purpose flour (use half whole wheat flour if desired)
⅔ cup sugar
4 teaspoons baking powder
2 teaspoons Chinese five-spice powder
Zest of 1 medium-size orange
1½ cups freshly squeezed orange juice
2 tablespoons canola oil
1 large egg
1 cup roughly chopped unsalted macadamia nuts

1. Preheat the oven to 350°F. Coat a 9-inch loaf pan with cooking spray. Set aside.

2. In a large bowl, combine the flour, sugar, baking powder, Chinese five-spice powder, and orange zest.

2. In another bowl, mix together the orange juice, oil, and egg. Mix well.

3. Make a well in the center of the flour mixture. Add the orange juice mixture and mix well but do not overbeat. The batter will be lumpy. Fold in the nuts. Pour the batter into the prepared loaf pan.

4. Bake for 45 minutes to 1 hour, until a cake tester inserted in the center comes out clean. Remove the pan from the oven and allow the bread to cool in the pan for 10 minutes. Turn out the bread from the pan onto a cooling rack and let cool completely.

Asian Pears with Lemony Herbs

10 SERVINGS/SERVING SIZE: ½ CUP

PREPARATION TIME: 15 MINUTES

COOK TIME: 18 MINUTES

Take advantage of any lemony herbs you can find to enhance this skillet dessert. The pistachios provide a very welcome crunch and this hot dessert is lovely on a crisp winter day.

● ● ● ● ● ● ● ● ●

2 medium-size Asian pears, or 2 large Bosc pears
   Juice of ½ lemon
4 medium-size oranges
2 tablespoons unsalted butter
3 tablespoons brown sugar
2 tablespoons chopped toasted unsalted pistachios
2 tablespoons shredded fresh lemon thyme, lemon verbena, lemon basil, or lemon balm

1. Peel, core, and slice the pears into ¼-inch slices. Sprinkle the pears with the lemon juice to prevent browning and set aside.

2. Peel three of the oranges and remove all the white pith. Separate the oranges into sections. Juice the remaining orange and set aside.

3. Melt the butter in a large skillet over medium heat. Add the sugar and stir until dissolved. Add the pears and cook for 3 to 4 minutes per side, just until tender. Add the oranges and orange juice to the pan and cook for 1 to 2 minutes. Coat the fruit with the pan juices.

4. Use a slotted spoon to remove the pears and oranges from the syrup and place in a decorative bowl. Boil the juices remaining in the pan and reduce by one-fourth. Pour the juices over the fruit and garnish with pistachios and lemon herb of choice.

BASIC NUTRITIONAL VALUES

Calories 100
   Calories from Fat 30
Total Fat 3.5 g
   Saturated Fat 1.5 g
   Trans Fat 0 g
Cholesterol 5 mg
Sodium 0 mg
Total Carbohydrate 18 g
   Dietary Fiber 4 g
   Sugars 14 g
Protein 1 g

Plums with Cinnamon and Cloves

4 SERVINGS/SERVING SIZE: 1 PARCEL

PREPARATION TIME: 25 MINUTES

COOK TIME: 20 MINUTES

Baking *en papillote* (wrapped in parchment paper) is not just limited to main dish entrées. Making these bundles creates a juicy and spicy mix of flavors with plums as the focal point. You can try this recipe with peaches or nectarines as well.

✿ ✿ ✿ ✿ ✿ ✿ ✿ ✿

BASIC NUTRITIONAL VALUES

Calories 185
  Calories from Fat 65
Total Fat 7.0 g
  Saturated Fat 2.0 g
  Trans Fat 0 g
Cholesterol 10 mg
Sodium 0 mg
Total Carbohydrate 32 g
  Dietary Fiber 3 g
  Sugars 27 g
Protein 2 g

8 large black plums, pitted and sliced thickly
1 tablespoon unsalted butter
4 cinnamon sticks
8 whole cloves
4 tablespoons pure maple syrup
1 tablespoon fresh orange zest
  Juice of 1 orange
3 tablespoons toasted unsalted pecans

CLOVES

Cloves are the unopened and dried flower buds of an evergreen tree. The essential oil extracted from cloves contains a high percentage of eugenol. Eugenol soothes toothaches and is used in dental anesthetics. In many countries, cloves are chewed to relieve toothaches.

1. Preheat the oven to 400°F. Have ready four large pieces of parchment paper. In the center of each piece of parchment paper, place one-quarter of the plums, butter, cinnamon sticks, and cloves. Drizzle the plums with the maple syrup, orange zest, and orange juice.

2. Bring the two opposite ends of one piece of parchment paper together and fold over three times. Fold over the other ends twice and then tuck them underneath to form a parcel. Repeat to form the other four bundles.

3. Place all the parcels on a rimmed baking sheet. Bake for 20 minutes.

4. Remove the parcels from the oven and transfer carefully to individual plates. Carefully open each parcel and sprinkle with pecans.

Saffron and Vanilla Roasted Pears

8 SERVINGS/SERVING SIZE: ½ CUP

PREPARATION TIME: 20 MINUTES

COOK TIME: 20 MINUTES

Saffron typically appears in savory dishes; here I combine it with vanilla and cinnamon to create this fiber-rich dessert that has beautiful color and decadent taste.

● ● ● ● ● ● ● ●

1 small pinch of fresh saffron threads
4 tablespoons hot water
2 tablespoons unsalted butter, melted
1 tablespoon Marsala wine
1 tablespoon honey
½ teaspoon pure vanilla extract
¼ teaspoon ground cinnamon
4 large Bosc pears, unpeeled, sliced into ½-inch slices

1. Line two large baking sheets with parchment paper and set aside. Heat a small, dry skillet over medium-high heat. Add the saffron threads and toast for 30 seconds, until fragrant. Place the saffron threads in a mortar and pestle and crush the threads. Add the hot water and stir well.

2. Transfer the saffron liquid to a large bowl. Add the butter, Marsala wine, honey, vanilla, and cinnamon. Mix well. Add the sliced pears and toss to coat. Cover and let marinate for 30 minutes, during which time preheat the oven to 450°F.

3. Spread the pears on the baking sheets in one layer.

4. Roast the pears for 20 to 25 minutes, turning them over halfway through the cooking time, until the pears are soft and browned.

BASIC NUTRITIONAL VALUES

Calories 100
  Calories from Fat 25
Total Fat 3.0 g
  Saturated Fat 2.0 g
  Trans Fat 0 g
Cholesterol 10 mg
Sodium 0 mg
Total Carbohydrate 20 g
  Dietary Fiber 4 g
  Sugars 14 g
Protein 0 g

Lemon Thyme Fruit Salad

8 SERVINGS/SERVING SIZE: ½ CUP

PREPARATION TIME: 12 MINUTES

COOK TIME: 0

This fresh fruit salad is so refreshing on a hot day. This is a perfect example of layering flavors; lemon thyme and lemon zest different flavor intensities. Together, they produce this delightful healthy and lemony dessert.

⬥ ⬥ ⬥ ⬥ ⬥ ⬥ ⬥ ⬥

BASIC NUTRITIONAL VALUES

Calories 100
  Calories from Fat 20
Total Fat 2.5 g
  Saturated Fat 0 g
  Trans Fat 0 g
Cholesterol 0 mg
Sodium 20 mg
Total Carbohydrate 19 g
  Dietary Fiber 2 g
  Sugars 15 g
Protein 3 g

1 medium-size Granny Smith apple, unpeeled, cored, and chopped
1 medium-size Gala apple, unpeeled, cored, and chopped
½ cup halved red grapes
½ cup halved green grapes
¼ cup raisins

Dressing
1 cup low-fat lemon yogurt
1 tablespoon finely minced fresh lemon thyme
2 teaspoons freshly squeezed lemon juice
2 teaspoons freshly squeezed orange juice
2 teaspoons honey
1 teaspoon lemon or orange zest

Garnish
¼ cup toasted slivered almonds

1. In a large bowl, combine the apples, grapes, and raisins.

2. Whisk together the dressing ingredients and pour over the fruit. Toss to coat. Top each serving with slivered almonds.

THYME
Since ancient times, thyme has been used, not only for its aroma and flavor, but also for its medicinal properties. Thymol, an essential oil extracted from thyme, is a natural antiseptic, antispasmodic, and expectorant. Thymol is frequently used as an ingredient in many over-the-counter cough syrups. A cup of thyme tea is believed to help relieve cough symptoms.

In the Middle Ages, thyme was placed underneath pillows to ward off nightmares and aid sleep. Diluted thyme oil applied to the soles of the foot is believed to prevent snoring and aid in sleeping.

Strawberry Lemon Granita

8 SERVINGS/SERVING SIZE: ½ CUP

PREPARATION TIME: 10 MINUTES

COOK TIME: 0

Refreshing on any hot summer day, this lightly lemon-infused berry granita hits the spot. Just be patient with the process of freezing the strawberries and don't be afraid to scrape really hard to create the ice crystals. Better than ice pops and certainly lower in calories than ice cream, granitas are sophisticated for the few ingredients required.

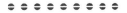

1 cup water

⅓ cup sugar

2 sprigs fresh lemon verbena or lemon thyme, or 1 teaspoon dried

1 (2-inch) piece fresh lemon zest

3 cups washed and hulled fresh strawberries

1. In a small saucepan, heat the water over medium heat until hot but not boiling. Add the sugar, herbs, and lemon zest. Let cool to room temperature. Strain and discard the fresh herbs and lemon zest.

2. Puree the berries in a food processor or blender. Slowly pour in the syrup and blend well.

3. Pour the strawberry puree into a 9 by 13-inch baking dish. Freeze the pan for about 20 minutes. Using a fork, scrape the frozen sections on the outer edges of the pan into the center of the pan. Freeze the mixture again for 20 minutes. Scrape the puree again. Repeat this process every 20 minutes until the liquid is frozen into flaky crystals with a sorbetlike consistency.

4. Serve immediately. To serve, scrape the granita into individual dessert dishes and top with a leaf of fresh lemon verbena.

BASIC NUTRITIONAL VALUES

Calories 50

    Calories from Fat 0

Total Fat 0.0 g

    Saturated Fat 0 g

    Trans Fat 0 g

Cholesterol 0 mg

Sodium 0 mg

Total Carbohydrate 13 g

    Dietary Fiber 1 g

    Sugars 11 g

Protein 0 g

Lavender Biscotti

MAKES 4 DOZEN SMALL
BISCOTTI/SERVING SIZE: 2 BISCOTTI

PREPARATION TIME: 25 MINUTES

COOK TIME: 50 MINUTES

A friend of mine, Ellen Toups, who loves to fiddle with unusual herbs and spices and is a fabulous baker, came up with this dreamy, heavenly scented biscotti. This has a delightful but strong flavor of lavender. If you prefer something milder, reduce the lavender or use herbes de Provence, which contains just a little lavender.

* * * * * * * *

2¼	cups all-purpose flour
1	teaspoon baking powder
½	teaspoon baking soda
⅔	cup sugar
3	large eggs
3	tablespoons clover honey
1	teaspoon pure vanilla extract
1	tablespoon fresh orange zest
1	tablespoon dried culinary-grade lavender blossoms

1. Preheat the oven to 350°F. Place the oven rack in the middle of the oven. Cover a large baking sheet with parchment paper and set aside. Sift the flour, baking powder, and baking soda into a small bowl.

2. In a large bowl, whisk the sugar and eggs to a light lemon color and stir in the honey, vanilla extract, orange zest, and lavender. Sift the dry ingredients over the egg mixture and then fold in until the dough is just combined. Do not overmix.

3. Mold half the dough into a 3-inch-wide log on the prepared baking sheet. Do the same with the remaining dough. Flour your hands, quickly stretch each portion of dough into a rough 13 by 2-inch log, placing the logs about 3 inches apart on the cookie sheet. Pat each dough log to smooth it. Bake, turning the pan around once about halfway through the baking time, until the loaves are golden and just beginning to crack on top, about 35 minutes.

4. Remove the biscotti from the oven and lower the oven temperature to 325°F. Let the loaves cool on the pan for 10 to 15 minutes. Use a serrated knife to cut each loaf diagonally into ⅜-inch slices.

5. Lay the slices about ½ inch apart on the cookie sheet, cut side up, and return them to the oven. Bake for 7 to 8 minutes. Turn over each cookie and bake for another 7 to 8 minutes, until the biscotti are crisp and golden brown on both sides. Transfer the biscotti to a wire rack and let cool completely. Biscotti can be stored in an airtight container for up to one month.

BASIC NUTRITIONAL VALUES

Calories 80
  Calories from Fat 5
Total Fat 0.5 g
  Saturated Fat 0 g
  Trans Fat 0 g
Cholesterol 25 mg
Sodium 50 mg
Total Carbohydrate 17 g
  Dietary Fiber 0 g
  Sugars 8 g
Protein 2 g

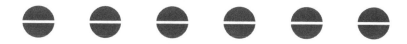

Appendix: Menus

Southwestern BBQ

Tomato Corn Salsa (page 29)

Tequila Lime Chicken (page 72)

Southwestern Coleslaw (page 104)

Chocolate Chile Nut Meringues (page 144)

• • • • • • • • • •

Indian-Style Light Lunch

Potato Pockets (page 30)

Indian Lentil Soup (page 125)

Baked Apples with Garam Masala (page 151)

• • • • • • • • • •

Easy Family Dinner

Zesty Oven-Fried Chicken (page 75)

Steak Fries (page 102)

Chopped Vegetable Salad with Garlic Herb Dressing (page 105)

Plums with Cinnamon and Cloves (page 155)

Time to Impress

Star Anise Cold Blueberry Soup (page 140)

Sichuan Lamb (page 79)

*Beet, Carrot, and Daikon Salad with Ginger Five Spice Dressing
(page 115)*

Chinese Five-Spice Fruit Kebabs (page 149)

• • • • • • • • • •

Brunch Celebration

Herb Frittata (page 82)

Cherry Tomato and Avocado Salad (page 94)

Fennel and Orange Salad (page 101)

Apple Thyme Upside-Down Cake (page 146)

• • • • • • • • • •

Caribbean Night

Caribbean-Style Pork Tenderloin with Melon Salsa (page 62)

Caribbean Sweet Potatoes (page 118)

green salad

Caribbean Citrus Pineapple (page 145)

• • • • • • • • • •

Be My Valentine

Italian Roasted Red Pepper Soup with Garlic Croutons (page 124)

Classic Steak au Poivre (page 81)

Linguine with Walnuts and Garlic and Herbs (page 97)

Simply Roasted Garlic Asparagus (page 116)

Berries in Ginger Peppercorn Syrup (page 148)

Ladies' Lunch

Lemon Pepper Shrimp Skewer with Grape Tomato Relish (page 24)

Zuppa di Ceci (page 127)

Goat Cheese Penne with Garlic and Herbs (page 90)

Watercress and Radicchio Salad (page 119)

Lavender Biscotti (page 159)

• • • • • • • • • •

The Big Game

Tuscan White Bean Dip (page 45)

Guacamole (page 40)

Garlic and Herb Pita Chips (page 46)

Chipotle Chips (page 47)

Veal and Mushroom Stew (page 139)

Haricots Verts with Cherry Tomatoes (page 107)

Lemon Thyme Fruit Salad (page 157)

• • • • • • • • • •

Summer Dinner on the Patio

Roasted Italian Edamame (page 25)

Lemon Pepper Turkey Burgers (page 70)

Grilled Italian Plum Tomatoes (page 110)

Herbes de Provence Squash (page 109)

Strawberry Lemon Granita (page 158)

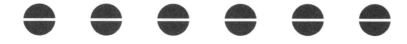

Acknowledgments

They say a writer's life can be a lonely one. But in my case as a cookbook writer, it is anything but! In fact one of my favorite things about cookbooks is the wonderful collaboration you can have with so many great people. Indeed, cookbook writing is all about teamwork.

There are many people to thank on my team. First, is Katie McHugh of Da Capo Press for another fabulous opportunity to write for you. Thank you for your strong belief that a deliciously designed low-sodium cookbook is not only current but a need that had to be fulfilled. Thank you for letting me fill that spot!

To my super agent Beth Shepard of Beth Shepard Communications, LLC, who has stood by for so many years, through project after project and who knew that this low-sodium cookbook could make a true and lasting difference to so many people who need flavor sans the salt. Her suggestions and guidance are truly my shining light.

To the incredible and ultra creative team of my photographer Renee Comet and food stylist Lisa Cherkasky, who give my food the true meaning of *mouthwatering*. I know I am fortunate to be the recipient of their perfection and the exacting quality of their work.

While first and foremost my recipes need to be delicious, they also need to be nutritionally sound. My utmost thanks goes to my longtime nutrition analyst, Madelyn Wheeler, MS, RD, FADA, CD, whose efficiency in preparing each recipe's nutrition profile is consistently accurate. I always appreciate her guidance on how to design recipes keeping the health of my readers as top priority.

No recipe just goes from my lips to print. A whole team of expert testers taste every single recipe and I am proud to have these fine women and men as part of my regular cookbook testing staff. Kudos go to Anna Berman, Olga Berman, Pam Braun, Michele Dalton, Amanda Markulec, Scott Naples, Kathy Pandol, Kristina Razon, Wendy Stuart who also contributed recipes, Paige Weaver and Maria Zebrowski. Their tireless efforts never go unnoticed.

My many thanks to Andy Bellatti, RD, who served as the books research associate. I am always impressed by Andy's relentless search to separate nutrition fact from fiction and I am truly grateful for our partnership. Nothing ever gets by Andy without a "real grilling" of the truth; this is what our nutrition industry is certainly challenged to find daily.

To some truly fabulous colleagues who contributed healthy, tasty recipes. I love that we can all share in spreading the word that low sodium can taste great. My thanks to Emma Stirling, APD; Ellen Toups; Danielle Turner; Jill Weisenberger, RD; and Diane Welland, RD.

And finally, a big hats-off to two people who were my right hands on this book, Ramzi Faris and Cecilia Stoute. They managed the testing teams so smoothly and coordinated the paperwork necessary to pull this cookbook together. I truly could not have done it without them both and to them I am eternally indebted.

—*Robyn Webb*

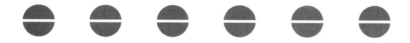

Index